BOTCHED

SETH LARREN

True Cases of Horrific

Medical Errors, Negligence,

and A Survivor's Story

Legal Disclaimer & Terms of Use

Today, there is marginal discussion about tort reform and medical malpractice lawsuits. These discussions convey varying opinions on where to cast blame and how the problem can best be corrected. In this book, the author adds his own view to the discussion by providing an exclusive perspective of personal observation.

Every attempt has been made to validate information provided in this publication; however, neither the author nor the publisher assumes any responsibility for errors, omissions, or contrary interpretation of the subject matter herein. Under no circumstance will any blame or legal responsibility be held against the publisher or author for any damages, reparation, or monetary loss due to the information contained within this book, either directly or indirectly. Case summaries recorded in this book are of public record, have been reviewed and verified, complete with case numbers as available. These cases are all included to substantiate evidence that medical negligence cases are real, tragic events affecting real people. These cases are verifiable through public access records. In a conscious effort to retain vital accuracy of each case presented in *Botched*, actual city/state locations where the specific injury occurred along with the name of hospital, clinic, medical center, or treatment facility have not been changed.

Out of respect for the victims of medical injury and their families, regarding all the other cases within, the author has voluntarily altered the names of individual plaintiffs and their respective families. Individual defendant names have also been altered in a spirit of professional courtesy and to avoid potential legal challenges from these parties.

Excluding the author's own malpractice case, all other cases presented inside this book have already been concluded, complete with a jury verdict or pre-court settlement. The inclusion of these cases will have no effect on the outcome of any of them or the author's case. Regarding the author's personal story, the names of all treating physicians, medical facilities, centers, and clinics have been voluntarily altered due to the pending outcome of the author's case. With respect to the surgeons, doctors and nurses who worked to repair the damage done to his spouse, the author offers his sincere gratitude to these exemplary professionals, acknowledging the benefit they serve in their field.

Please note the information contained within this document is for educational and recreational purposes only. All effort has been made to ensure the information is accurate, reliable, and competent. No guarantees of any kind are declared or implied. Reader acknowledges that the author is not engaging in the rendering of legal, financial, medical, or professional advice. Though he has learned plenty through his experience and personal research, in matters pertaining to doctors, hospitals, medical staff personnel, lawyers, litigation, financial or personal matters, the author does not claim to be an expert. Therefore, any conclusions put forth by the author are his opinions and should not be used as expert, legal or professional advice. If you, a relative or someone else you know is currently being treated by a physician for any illness, listen to your doctor and follow treatment recommendations. In the event you find yourself at odds with your doctor regarding any medical matter, please make every effort to obtain a second opinion from another physician. Never totally remove yourself from a doctor's care for anything you are currently being treated for. There is never a good reason to refuse medical services or deny yourself from seeing a physician when you could likely benefit from such care. Do not hesitate to seek a licensed medical professional if your condition dictates such attention and care.

Amy

Although the past was difficult, you somehow managed to work through it all with fortitude and supernatural strength. You undoubtedly beat the odds, defied expectations and epitomized strength, courage, and determination through a very difficult process. Your incredibly miraculous recovery has taught me much while solidifying my commitment to you and to our marriage.

CONTENTS

INTRODUCTION

As a man who appreciates the many wonders of science, I marvel at the extraordinary capabilities of modern medical science. The ability of a micro-surgeon to reattach a severed limb to working functionality it is nothing short of amazing. When one considers the vast complexity of the human body and factors in all the variables that can go wrong in trying to repair it, it is truly a wonder that success is more the expected outcome than failure. Medical science is an interesting field and the modern advancements of medicine enhance the quality of life for all people who are successfully treated through these methods.

With all the advancements of modern medicine, there is, on occasion, moments when error in medical treatment can cause severe injury to the patient, thereby resulting in a painful and life-changing experience for the victim, the victim's family and loved ones. This is not the norm, but it does happen. Living through such an event can give one an entirely new perspective on the medical profession, and tactics used by the medical establishment to fight or dissuade legal recourse after a medical injury has occurred is every bit as astonishing as any wonder of modern medical science. Beyond the medical injury, the legal war that pursues reveals a dark side of medicine of which few know exist. *Botched* exposes the negative side of the patient-physician relationship once medical intervention goes sour.

In his book, *"First, Do No Harm"*, board-certified surgeon, Dr. Ira E. Williams, makes a magnificent appeal to those in his profession, after admitting to the "deeply entrenched conspiracy of silence among doctors and medical personnel." He compellingly makes the case how doctors interpret the Hippocratic Oath as, "Do no harm, but if you do, keep your mouth shut."

Medical malpractice lawsuits occur fewer times than one might imagine, yet, with somewhere between 90,000 to 200,000 annual medical malpractice deaths, overall medical negligence occurrences are far more frequent than the number of lawsuits suggests. Some make it to court and others never will. One thing is for sure: of all medical injury complaints that make it to court, many are justifiable when one examines the details and specifics.

Many of us have heard of a scenario where a surgeon operated on the wrong appendage, a patient died from being given the wrong drug or a nurse fails to carry out plan-of-care orders, all resulting in negative consequences for the patient. When we hear about such incidents it isn't likely that we hear the details surrounding these cases. Case details insinuate errors such as these are avoidable, occurring primarily due to oversight or carelessness.

The widely held belief about medical malpractice lawsuits is that they are simply frivolous complaints launched with the malicious intent of "striking it rich" at the expense of some unwary doctor. In my discovery I have found this to be far from true. In many cases – and this is certainly true in my own malpractice case – the victim will often be reluctant to go the legal route, allowing the offending practitioner tremendous leeway in efforts to preserve the treatment relationship with their doctor. Still, politicians echo the popular belief of malpractice frivolity and use it as a basis for limiting awards to injured individuals who are the true victims of bad medicine. The so-called tort reform legislation feeds this erroneous belief by looping all malpractice complaints into a single award-cap limit, sending the message that health care providers are the victims rather than those who are physically injured because of bad medical care.

Like most other issues, when it comes to the topic of medical malpractice there are two primary positions one can take. The first position is one that leans in favor of the medical industry, primarily the doctors, hospitals, insurance, and pharmaceutical companies, along with health care administrators and pro-medical politicians, who basically believe that there are too many malpractice lawsuits, and they are the primary contributor to overall and increasing health care costs. The second position is that of the victim, their loved ones, and their attorneys, who hold the position that poor medical care, doctors who provide substandard care, profit-prioritizing insurance companies, medical treatment of illegal aliens, and government regulation are the key reasons costs in the medical industry are so astronomical, and that these costs can be better controlled when these matters are specifically addressed. Whichever position one might hold, there is some truth to either of these sides.

In years past, the medical community has long enjoyed the position of prestige, where medical professionals and authorities in the field were regarded as warriors for the good of public health. More recently, the medical industry has come under rare and critical scrutiny – not necessarily by the media, but primarily by the public. This is due, in part, to authorities within the medical community's assertions and response to the COVID-19 pandemic, where much of the recommendations were not grounded in scientific fact, but rather, hype and ineffective appeasement antics that arguably caused more harm than good.

Medical authorities lied about the source of the COVID-19 infection, kept changing their suggestions on how to protect against contracting coronavirus, ultimately taking up a militant stance against those who dared questioned them. The *science factor* of the medical community's response to COVID-19 was secondary to the primary politicization of the disease. Masks became a symbol of submission, giving people a false sense of protection against transmission of the disease. Overpaid medical bureaucrats, with the help of the media, were not only participants in the hysteria, but instigators of it. Pharmaceutical companies trotted out a minimally tested, two-phase shot that they dubbed as a "vaccine" which turned out to be nothing more than a wishful panacea, requiring recipients to keep getting boosters that seemed just as ineffective as the initial dose shots. People who resisted being forced to get a shot were villainized and targeted for ridicule and prosecution, with many folks losing their jobs and careers. The community began targeting individuals within their own industry who didn't jump through the hoops and tow the authoritative line. The universal blanket approach to force everyone to receive the shots, without regard to any other medical factor or condition, forced the public to finally wise up to the silliness surrounding the hype. In this, the notion of "do no harm" took an intentional back seat as the medical community, pharmaceutical industry and indeed, the government itself (as it imposed its overreaching mandates on everyone) all became a picture of a dystopian reality where tyrants impose their irrational will and authority on its lowly subjects.

Additionally, the medical industry is receiving much needed scrutiny for its inhumane involvement in this crazy transgenderism propaganda infecting the nation. Medical practitioners are dishing out life-altering, transition-mutilation surgeries and supplying development hormone blockers to minors who have no idea that they are simply pawns in an immoral social and political scheme. For the recipients of this barbaric version of "medicine", they are – in many cases – receiving irreversible treatment that will relegate them to an unfulfilling life – all for the sake of an industry that has chosen to prioritize a few bucks over the total value of a human life. We've seen this preference of financial materialism over human dignity metastasize first in the abortion industry. As the value of human life diminished in the womb, we now see it diminishing outside of the womb in the form of transgenderism. Rather than dealing medically with the mental health issues these poor individuals are obviously suffering from, the practitioners would instead prefer to prioritize their "professional" earnings over the value and quality of life of their human patients who rely on them for their professional expertise.

These are just a couple of examples where the medical industry is in outright violation of its Hippocratic Oath. Admittedly however, because I am not educated in medicine, it is a bit outside the scope of my ability to give equal weight to both sides (either in favor of or against) of the medical malpractice debate, so I will not attempt to do so. My perspective comes from one who has experienced the dark side of medicine.

Despite popular belief about medical malpractice claims, existing laws in most states lean heavily in favor of the medical practitioners, making it very tough for those persons injured negligently to successfully pursue legal damages. From the onset, malpractice victims face a steep uphill battle trying to get their case through discovery and into court. Since I personally know this to be true, *Botched* is written in support of the second position of the medical malpractice debate – on behalf of the injured party. The patient perspective is the position from where I feel adequate to write on medical malpractice. To date I have yet to find an adequate book written on the topic, almost as if there is some unwritten rule discouraging open debate on the matter. Regardless, it is my hope that this book can help anyone who finds himself/herself in the unfortunate circumstance resulting from a medical injury.

Through personal experience I know that a malpractice injury can often be an indefinite, ongoing matter for the victim while the offending practitioner can continue to practice medicine on other unsuspecting patients, even before a resolution is reached.

While the victim struggles in recovery through the physical pain, emotional distress and psychological scars left from the medical injury, the practitioner can mentally put the incident behind them and continue work as if nothing significant occurred.

It is conceivable that for every point I make in support of the injured victim of medical negligence, a counterpoint can be made against the same in favor of the physicians and other medical practitioners. Recognizing this, I have chosen against attempting to proportionately cover both sides of the malpractice argument in this book. I discuss the medical malpractice issue in a truthful manner solely from my experience, yet I am not really trying to be balanced. Someone more qualified than I can write in defense of the medical community regarding malpractice. My whole purpose in being forthcoming about my position in this malpractice debate is to prevent any misconceptions about the way the subject matter is presented in *Botched*. If my honesty is in question, then the words in this book are pointless.

One may wonder why anybody would write on such a contentious topic as medical injuries and malpractice cases. Is this some slick scheme or political effort to weigh in on relating policy issues? And if not, why else would anyone opt to publish their story of a failed medical procedure?

Well, honestly, I am not political in the sense that I am an activist. I am not a left-wing democrat. To the contrary, I am a conservative who votes republican and a card-carrying member of the GOP. But those whom I support politically aren't necessarily on my side on the medical malpractice issue. In fact, I suppose their position on the matter of tort law is based solely on politics. Be that as it may, it may be difficult to understand any reason one would write about medical malpractice.

It was only a few years earlier that my wife, Amy, endured a life-threatening injury from a botched medical procedure. During her recovery era I often found myself angry as I watched her struggle daily to get through it. It diminished her quality of life and I lost much of her companionship through the recovery period. Highly frustrated in our situation, I kept wondering how many other people had faced something similar. If a medical injury could happen to us, then certainly it is probable there are others who lived through some form of medical injury. In my search to find supporting literature to help me through the fear, the anger and convoluted legal process, I soon realized the scarcity of substance-oriented material on this topic.

It was a tough decision for me to write this book because it tells of events that are most personal in every way. This was a time of extraordinary pain, grief, and slow, diligent recovery. It was a Dark Age period in our life where forward progress was almost nonexistent. The ripple-effect of my wife's medical injury still affects us today and probably will many more years to come. These are matters that normally one would only share with immediate family members, the closest of friends or clergy. Yet, the longer I thought about it the more I realized that what my wife survived was *anything* but normal. This story deserves to be told, even at the risk of alienating several personal friends and acquaintances who are members of the medical profession. Considering the incredible nature of our story this is a risk that I have come to accept.

After struggling in my decision to write this book, I next had to determine how much information I wanted to reveal to protect my family and myself from ridicule or incidents that might arise from this book's release. Changes in the names of individuals, certain medical entities and specific injury information regarding my wife had to be taken into consideration. I chose to reveal as much factual information as necessary to adequately tell our story, though I have intentionally removed the year pertaining to events happening in our personal story. Also, names of all individual medical personnel involved have been voluntarily altered for obvious reasons. Physicians of whom I felt have proactively positioned themselves against our pending malpractice case will also get the benefit of a pseudo identity.

Once determined I was going to complete the book and publish it, I soon learned that writing can be a laboring endeavor. The best writing happens when the author works hard to communicate his message rather than the reader struggling to understand it. In *Botched*, my difficulty in trying to communicate my message lay in the challenge of simplicity regarding medical procedures and terminology. Keeping in mind that I wanted this book to be more for the public than the medical community, I've tried to write it in a style that will appeal to people unfamiliar with the medical or legal world, even though most of what this book is about encompasses both.

Without question, I absolutely love my wife. Certainly, she is much stronger than those who know her give her credit for. She is kind, gentle, original, and placed aside her own personal concerns of privacy for the benefit of other medical malpractice victims. She has lost much, and somehow turned that physical loss into a tremendous spiritual asset. We can all learn from her tenacity and selflessness, for it is with her approval and support that we are honored to share this very personal story. And as you read it, I ask that you do so with an open mind and without judgment, extending to us the courtesy of empathy and the benefit of non-perversion. It isn't easy opening up one's life in a book for the world to read but we chose to do so to help others and communicate the "other side" of the medical malpractice debate.

While critical of the medical community in the scope of a malpractice situation, this book was not intentionally written to discredit the medical profession – heaven knows we need good, educated, and qualified specialists in the medical business. Truly, if there were more good doctors and a self-policing system within the medical establishment to weed out careless ones, then this book might not be necessary. My purpose in writing this book is to expose the dark tactics employed by the medical industry and their attorneys during malpractice litigation, discuss the medical malpractice lawsuit process, summarize a few cases where malpractice lawsuits were found in favor of the injured party and share our personal story.

As a former non-medical hospital administrative employee, I have some insight into the medical environment than those persons not affiliated with the industry. Still, I do not consider myself to be a member of the medical community. I am not an attorney and make no claim to be an expert on the issue of medical malpractice. The sole reference from which I write is that of someone whose spouse has experienced the random misfortune of a botched surgery – an event which led to a situation where I had no choice except to hire attorneys. I feel these experiences qualify me to write on the matter of medical negligence, because in addition to the misfortune of living through a botched surgery as experienced by my wife, I have taken the time to do my homework on the subject. What I have discovered is both compelling and disturbing.

I will admit that in writing this book and reliving those moments of Amy's pain, suffering and struggles, I found myself going through periods of searing anger – anger I couldn't let myself feel when she was hospitalized. I will also confess that the further I progressed in writing our story I discovered that doing so had become therapeutic for me, perhaps because I was finally recording everything. Strangely, writing about what happened has forced me to grapple with a negative and turn it into a positive, and I hope this work will become an ally to any person who finds themselves in the terrible midst of a medical malpractice situation. It is also my hope that this book will provide a different perspective for state legislatures and Congress in future tort reform debates.

It may be possible that you know someone who is the victim of medical malpractice, or maybe that *someone* is you. If so, you know that the lives of those who have lived through a medical malpractice injury are changed forever: in some cases, for the better – but sadly, in many cases, for the worse. People who have lived through a medical injury know the feelings of fear, helplessness, anger, and resentment. Even after hiring an attorney, treading the murky legal waters of medical malpractice litigation can at times be very frustrating and humiliating, no matter how seemingly strong your case may appear. From my experience there are moments when you can feel as if no one cares about the horrible reality of your predicament and if you happen to be the spouse or guardian of the person injured, you will often question how and why the events leading up to the injury have occurred and if there was something you personally did to contribute to the injury.

These feelings are all expected and normal. However, it is imperative to understand that if you honestly trusted your physician and heeded the medical information and advice they provided before a medical injury has occurred, then truly, you are not to blame, even though the defense will use tactics to make it appear as if it was somehow your fault.

There may even be some feeling of embarrassment about pursuing a malpractice suit against a doctor. Why? Because of the stigma that is placed on those who try to obtain damages. There is a popular but unfounded belief that plaintiffs in a malpractice lawsuit have only one goal in mind which is striking it rich – but this is simply not true. The public is quite uneducated about this topic and the dynamics involved, and it is my hope to educate the public about this long, tedious process. There are many malpractice cases out there that deserve to be tried in court, so if you are the victim of a botched surgery or another form of medical malpractice, as you read through the pages of this book, please take some comfort in knowing that you are not alone.

CHAPTER 1

Day 16: March 22 – 1:55 PM

It was just before 2:00 in the afternoon on March 22nd, when I arrived home with my wife, Amy. We were both very grateful to have made it here together, as things could have turned out much differently. While we recognized there would be tremendous challenges ahead for us over the next few months, little did we know that these efforts would be even greater than the one she had just overcame.

While in the hospital I didn't really ponder the challenge daily life would be for Amy once she was discharged and how these challenges would impact us. My initial focus was on getting her well enough to come home and I hadn't realized how our life would kick into survival mode for the next several months after her discharge. Somehow, I expected that with having Amy home, recovery would be a downhill effort. But the days ahead would prove that the real fight was just beginning, while at the same time challenge our marriage in ways no newlywed couple should have to face.

We were arriving home from the hospital where Amy had just spent 16 grueling days, 7 of which were in intensive care. She was unconscious for the first 4½ days, sedated due to the severity of major injuries sustained while being treated by surgeons and medical doctors. This condition was the result of a botched surgery – a surgery that was supposed to have been a routine outpatient procedure. Unfortunate for us, there was nothing routine about the procedure.

Amy's frail body was incredibly weak from trauma and the subsequent surgeries she had survived. Her weight at discharge was a mere 80 pounds, about 25 pounds under her regular weight. Even for her height of 5'4", she was skin and bones by anybody's standard. She was in a lot of pain but tried to hide the fact with a forced level of optimism. Though glad to arrive home to the familiar setting that she hadn't seen in about 2 weeks, the difficulties of life wouldn't wait a moment, not even from the time I first helped her exit the car.

Home for us was a decently furnished upstairs apartment. Everything in it was ours short of the major appliances. Getting Amy upstairs and inside our apartment was a prophetic moment for the days, weeks, and many months ahead. This was a trek that was not going to be easy.

Amy's injuries prevented her from being able to stand or walk without assistance. Per my request she was discharged with a folding aluminum walker, necessary for ambulation (walking) assistance due to her injuries. Even at this point we didn't know the full extent of those injuries, but the future would reveal the depth and scope of the physical damage, scars, and pain. Her discharge from the hospital was itself a milestone - the first of many.

Yet one of the doctors authorizing the discharge did not want to acknowledge the degree of Amy's injuries and resisted the idea of discharging her with a walker. In fact, this vascular surgeon who had operated on her twice apparently told one of the nurses that her inability to walk was a "mentally manifested" matter rather than actual, as if her lack of mobility was somehow a direct assault on his surgical ability. The attending nurse was upset with the surgeon for his lack of compassion and voiced her annoyance about this to Helen, my mother-in-law, whom would later inform me about it. What a pillar of arrogance and shallow character that this surgeon would respond so callously without ultimate regard for the patient. Amy's reality had nothing to do with his professional pride, and shame on him for discounting her pain. It wasn't as if he had to personally pay for the walker and it was pitiless of him to resist having it issued. Fortunate for him I didn't find out about his attitude *before* we left the hospital.

I removed Amy's walker from the back seat of the car and placed it right at the opened door on the passenger's side where she was seated. The back of the seat that she occupied was in a reclining position because it was too painful for her to sit upright. I encouraged her as I provided my hands and arms for assistance to help her up out of the vehicle. She slowly rose out of the seat as I helped her up. Once fully out of the car she grasped the handles of the walker, leaning her full weight on it as she began to inch forward to the base of the stairs of our apartment building.

Ascending the stairs was a task. I could only hold onto Amy gingerly because she had complained of aching and soreness of her extremities. She seemed to be able to cope with me holding onto the wrist of her arm that she placed around my neck. My other arm anchored around her small waist while her free hand held onto the stair rail. The walker remained behind us at the base of the stairs and as we began our ascent, it took slow and careful patience to get her up the steps successfully. From this task it was easy to see that the motions of this 23-year-old woman had become that of someone four times her age.

In her own car, Helen had followed us home from the hospital to help me carry in the many "get-well" gifts, flowers and other items that had accumulated during our residence at the hospital. Wanting to make sure that we made it home okay, Helen volunteered to stay with her daughter while I left to go to the pharmacy and have prescriptions filled. I was gone for a little over an hour; once I returned home my mother-in-law departed so that Amy would be able to rest.

Amy's nutritional intake was of immediate concern because she had lost quite a bit of weight and had issues with retaining and digesting food. The hospital's clinical dietician recommended Amy on a soft-food diet for this reason, so before returning home from the pharmacy I stopped to pick up a milkshake. She drank of it what she could, barely a third of the 22-ounce cup. If she were to gain her strength back she would have to improve at increasing her food consumption. Even this would be an obstacle for us.

This first day home was restless and problematic, a foretelling of the days ahead. Amy cried from post-operative pain, abdominal discomfort, soreness, and pain in her left leg, which was incredibly swollen. Her breathing was short and shallow. The hospital released her with a spirometer – an apparatus for measuring and strengthening her lung air capacity. She had to blow into the spirometer regularly, but whenever she blew into it the device indicated that she was barely managing half of the normal air capacity she should be able to generate from her lungs.

That evening Amy reached a point where she wanted to get out of her clothes so that she could take a shower. Her deep laceration wounds required us to prevent her from taking any baths for the time being. At the hospital, I was told that allowing her to sit in standing water for any length of time would cause the tissue around the wounds to soften and possibly reopen. It would also increase chances of infection. These concerns made sense to me, but the gynecologist who was responsible for Amy's surgical injury vehemently argued with the nurse who provided me this information. The nurse who told me that Amy should not take baths until permitted by the surgeon was simply repeating information the surgeon had told me previously. The gynecologist's position that Amy *could* take baths directly contradicted the surgeon's instructions. The nurse held her ground against the gynecologist, stating that in her entire nursing experience she had never heard of a patient with wounds like Amy's ever being allowed to take baths so soon after surgery. Neither relented on their opposing positions, but I was compelled to trust the advice of the surgeon and the nurse over the gynecologist's absurd position on the matter.

Because Amy could not stand on her own, I had to aid her in getting undressed and giving her the shower. It took some time for me to get her unclothed. Underneath her clothing were large, gauze bandages taped over the wounds on both sides of her ribcage and one side of her back. These bandages would have to be removed carefully, as tape holding on the bandages stuck to sensitive skin around her wounds. Every movement of her limbs caused her pain and she could only stand in a forward hunched-over position, not fully upright. Once I had removed the bandages, I was able to view for the first time all the incision wounds on her body absent of any covering. They were unpleasant to look at, to say the least.

A long major abdominal incision beginning at just below her sternum ran all the way down, around her navel and proceeded approximately five inches farther south. The length of this wound was a just over twelve inches. Another long incision – also approximately twelve inches long – began at the base of her right breast, extending and curving around her ribcage, ending on her back just below her right shoulder blade. Chest tube wounds, which are basically stab wounds, were present on both sides of her torso – two on the right, one on the left. There were wounds in the pelvic area on both sides. These awful scars would be the bane of countless sleepless nights, agonizing days, and lengthy, fruitless weekends.

Her left knee was swollen and protruded from a leg already thin from weight loss. This was an entirely mystery injury to us, but it caused Amy terrible pain, as did the laceration wounds on her upper body. In the days ahead she would suffer from intense headaches, nausea, bowel irregularity, body aches, shortness of breath, a growing resistance to the pain medicine, panic attacks, and the apparent onset of mild depression, probably caused by her sudden level of dependency and inability to move without pain and reduced capacity to ambulate.

In addition to these issues, Amy's right eye had sustained injury as well. The pupil was frozen small, and her iris did not respond to light even as her left eye appeared to function normally. The white area of her right eye was a tarnished, reddish-brown color and the eyelid drooped over her eye as if it were only half open. The injured eye looked dull and almost dead. Amy complained of blurred vision from this eye but did not realize how it had changed because she hadn't viewed a mirror since the very day she had entered the hospital. The condition of her right eye hinted of additional damage, far away from the lower pelvic and abdominal site where her original condition should have been confined.

I began the careful task of removing her clothing. The sweat-pant bottoms and t-shirt took longer to remove than I had expected. I helped her to put on a shower cap while she leaned on me for support. It required careful effort getting her into the shower where the warm water was already running, and there was no way to achieve this without my getting wet as well. The water from the shower head cascaded down her back as she leaned forward against the wall to help steady her balance. It would be less than 2 minutes before she signaled to get out, and as I helped her exit the shower, she cried from the discomfort that tormented her weak and frail body. Leaning on me again for balance, I managed to dry her off with a towel using a patting method. Once complete, I helped her get dressed into some loose shorts and a loose-fitting t-shirt. Stepping ever so slowly, the few feet from the bathroom to our bedroom where she would lay helplessly in pain for a number of days seemed further than I had ever noticed before. Upon reaching the bed, in a low and almost undistinguishable voice she asked for her pain medication.

Amy would be reliant on regular ample doses of hydrocodone (or 7.5mg Lortabs) every three to four hours. The good thing about the medicine was that it did have a side effect of drowsiness which probably aided her sleeping. But the negative side-effects were those of all narcotics: it could be habit forming and long-term use could result in liver damage. For now, these side-effect concerns would take a back seat to her priority need for comfort – to whatever extent this was feasible. The prescription helped her somewhat, but the duration of relief was very short for her.

After some time, Amy eventually drifted off to sleep, but the night would be a series of short naps rather than an overnight slumber. She woke up multiple times during the night sobbing from pain. Before her hospital stay, it was customary for her to sleep on her side, but as a result of the incision wounds from her surgeries, she could only manage to lie on her back. Lying on her sides put too much pressure against the wounds present on both sides of her torso. The agony she went through that first night at home was no improvement than when she was in the hospital. Her situation would get worse before it got better.

Every time Amy woke up that night, all I could do was talk to her and to let her know I was there. I repeatedly asked her to tell me what I could do to make her comfortable, but she wouldn't answer me – probably because she had no idea. I offered to take her back to a different hospital than the one she was discharged from and she absolutely refused. She was tired of hospitals and at that moment was fearful of doctors. There was a certain rationale to her fear, for the terrible condition she was presently in was far, far worse than any condition she had ever been in, and though she didn't know the extent of her injuries, she knew enough to recognize the fact that doctors were the cause of her current condition. Her fearful refusal to see a doctor would be the sole reason I delayed getting her back into a physician's office even though I felt she needed additional medical care.

For the next several days and even weeks, Amy's routine would be nothing more than a confinement to the bed or the sofa, interrupted only by trips to the bathroom. Since she could not walk without aid of the walker, getting to the bathroom and back to the sofa or bed was laboring and problematic. I assisted her at every opportunity and her existence would be a constant effort to manage pain while working on her ability to regain her appetite, increase her strength, and work on her breathing. Trying to ambulate without the walker was simply out of the question for the time being. She required close observation and there were times when family and friends would come by to sit with her in my absence.

It wasn't long after Amy's discharge from the hospital that my parents came from out of town to offer their assistance and company to her. Though my parents visited the hospital twice when Amy was hospitalized, this was the first time they had seen Amy since her discharge. Amy's deteriorated ability caused them to voice their concerns. My mother's reaction to Amy's situation was that of astonishment and disbelief as she commented that this shocking version of medicine ruined Amy's quality of life. Mom knew Amy would need special provisions to get by on a day-to-day basis and offered to take Amy home with her so that she could have continuous observation. My father's reaction was also one of astonishment and anger. My dad felt that the hospital releasing her in such poor shape was nothing short of criminal and he recommended that I admit her to another hospital so that she could fully recover before facing the challenges of daily living. Giving considerable attention to both suggestions, I concluded that Amy would benefit most by having me nearby.

We were all afraid of the possibility that Amy would never fully recover.

In Amy's and my decision to spend our life together, our plans for the future didn't really take into account the serious and disabling injuries that would befall her so soon after our vows, even though we promised each other companionship through circumstances better or worse – in sickness or health. Her injuries had affected us in many areas. Our immediate happiness would suffer, as well as our finances, our intimacy, our peace of mind, and our ability to trust the medical profession.

There was no lack of issues that surfaced in our life after Amy's hospitalization. Her hair turned lifelessly brittle due to the blood that had been left in it for days while she recovered in ICU. The hospital staff made no attempt to clean the blood out of her hair after surgery and from days of neglect the blood dried and matted her once beautiful brown hair. The lasting result of this oversight to clean her hair was breakage, hair loss, dullness and a total loss of vitality. Also, even though Amy always maintained excellent oral health, the huge amount of anesthesia she received for the surgeries became a catalyst to an erosion of tooth enamel and costly dental restoration services. The anesthesia was also believed to have played a role in the degradation of her hair. She ultimately became ashamed of her appearance and because of the disfiguring surgical scar running down the middle of her abdomen she vowed to never again wear a two-piece bathing suit or any clothing exposing her abdomen.

In the matter of our finances, the effect of Amy's injuries was an abrupt discontinuance of secondary income into our household – income that we were accustomed to having abruptly ceased. Amy pulled a nine-hour shift, working to 11:30 p.m. the night before her surgery. Since her discharge from the hospital, she could not go back to work. Her ability to get by each hour of every day without pain was a constant challenge that continuously defeated her. Her ability to walk was about as limited as that of a severely crippled person. With no immediate knowledge of whether this would be a temporary or permanent disability, her mental state was such that she didn't want to be around people, let alone in a work environment. These reasons prevented her from returning to work and our finances would soon compound upon us, adding an additional issue that would need attention.

As Amy's husband, I made every effort possible to be available to help her every step of the way. The issues she struggled with affected me too, more than I was willing to realize. Obviously, I didn't have to live through the physical pain she was experiencing but the significance of my inability to remove her discomfort bore down on me. I would have to learn to cope with the emotional challenges that something like this imposes. I was a young man who was overcome with mental fatigue and anxiety, resulting in my diagnosis of shingles – a very painful viral affliction usually effecting senior citizens but occasionally surfaces in younger people dealing with severe stress. Watching her in anguish tore at me because the nightmare of suffering through which Amy was experiencing would be something that I could not remove from her; this part of her predicament, she would have to work through individually, with me being there to assist as best I could.

Before Amy's medical injury and during the early period of her recovery, I was gainfully employed as an account manager for an office supply and technology company. My sales position eventually became a casualty of this injury upon our lives. Once the company's star salesman, life's immediate circumstances began to impact my performance and all the additional time off certainly didn't help matters. My time spent away from work vaporized all of my vacation time and paid personal leave. My work attendance fell, with my job performance taking a serious hit. To avoid inevitable termination, I voluntarily resigned – just to retain the last bit of dignity I had left. A good paying position would soon give way to mediocre jobs through temporary agency employment and overnight positions so my days could be open to drive Amy to therapy and accompany her to doctor office visits. There would be many.

The lasting result of this reduction in our income led to an accumulation of medical bills, unpaid debts, deterioration of our credit score and an embarrassing financial insult to the horrific injury. It would ripple into financial challenges that we had not prepared ourselves to encounter.

In the many days prior to Amy's botched surgery and extended hospitalization, there were certain events which happened that led us to the point where we were convinced (with help from the culprit gynecologist) that Amy needed to go through with the surgery. It had been our intent, hope and belief that Amy was getting the best care from her attending physician. But we were young and naïve. Our ignorance about such matters prevented us from recognizing that Amy was not receiving the best care this area of medicine had to offer. The events that happened along the way really tested the limits of human patience and tolerance.

To fully appreciate the degree of our malpractice complaint against Amy's former doctor – and possibly other involved practitioners – it is necessary to go back a few months earlier in our marriage and cover the events leading up to this moment where we were returning home from the hospital.

CHAPTER 2

July 18 (Eight Months Before March 7)

Amy and I were thrilled when we discovered that she was pregnant. We had married earlier in the summer and as a newly married couple, we were naturally quite optimistic about the possibility of a child becoming a part of our new life together. We sought out a local gynecologist to treat Amy through this exciting time. We did not seek any referral recommendations from family or friends for physician referral purposes. This was a personal decision that we wanted to be our own.

We had specific reasons for choosing the gynecologist we eventually ended up with.

First, the doctor had to be a member of our PPO insurance network. For the claims to be paid at the network rate the doctor needed to be a member. The good thing about this was that our insurance had a decent list of providers in our area of residence who were members. This gave us a large selection of doctors to choose from.

Second, the doctor had to be a *Medical Board-Certified Specialist*. It was our belief that a Board-Certified Specialist was the best of the best. We did not want to take any chances with a less qualified physician and so being a Board-Certified doctor was an important part of our selection criteria.

Third, it was important to Amy that the doctor be female. This was her preference and so it became mine as well. To her it was just a matter of comfort – and that was easily understandable to me.

Lastly, the doctor had to be within a reasonable distance from where we lived and fortunately for us our apartment at that time was within a mile of several medical offices, hospitals and clinics.

The doctor we ended up selecting met all our conditions, which Amy and I both liked.

"Dr. Keel" – as I will refer to her – was a Medical Board-Certified OB/gynecologist. We would see her for the first time ever only a few days after we learned of the pregnancy. Our first appointment with Dr. Keel confirmed Amy's pregnancy, a sonogram/ultrasound was performed, and we were able to see images of our developing baby. Amy was prescribed prenatal vitamins and provided a calendar, nutritional chart and other literature from which to track the progress of her pregnancy.

I attended most Amy's appointments with Dr. Keel. In fact, I believe I was present at them all. The thought of my wife having to go to these appointments alone didn't sit well with me and so I decided early on that I would attend as many of her office visits as I could.

During the second office visit to Dr. Keel's office, an ultrasound detected a weakening of our unborn baby's heart. We were told during that visit that the pregnancy was in jeopardy. Eventually we lost the baby. Shortly after miscarriage was diagnosed, Dr. Keel performed an outpatient gynecological procedure (D&C) on Amy to remove the residual fetal tissue from the uterus. It was a devastating blow for us, as Amy was about 11 weeks when she miscarried. Some time had passed. Amy and I determined we could get pregnant in the future and our lives soon returned to normal after the loss. The first D&C was performed In late summer of 20xx, just weeks after Amy and I were married. As far as I knew at the time, the D&C was performed as needed, without any issues or complications. We continued seeing Dr. Keel for all of Amy's medical matters in this area.

In a subsequent appointment with Dr. Keel, we were told by Dr. Keel that one of the earlier ultrasounds showed what appeared to be a bicornuate (irregular-shaped) uterus, and/or a uterine septum, which was described to us as thick tissue within the uterine wall. It was believed that this septum contributed to blockage of vital nutrition and other necessities for a baby to develop and grow within the womb. Dr. Keel persuaded us that the septum would have to be removed to improve Amy's chances of having a full-term pregnancy.

Dr. Keel discussed with us the need to further evaluate this uterine abnormality and recommended a hysterosalpingogram or an HSG (for short). The HSG is an x-ray test that examines the inside of the uterus, fallopian tubes and the surrounding area, often done in women who are unable to become pregnant. During an HSG, contrast dye is injected through a thin tube into the uterus through the pelvis. As contrast dye passes through the uterus and the fallopian tubes, x-ray pictures are taken, and the pictures can reveal injury, abnormal structure or blockage between the fallopian tube and the uterus. This was scheduled to take place sometime in December of that year.

Prior to this HSG procedure, in mid-November, Amy believed she had become pregnant again and a home pregnancy test showed a positive reading, but we wanted to be sure and sought confirmation from Dr. Keel's office before fully rejoicing in the news. Amy called and scheduled an appointment with Dr. Keel to verify the pregnancy. The appointment was made and attended by both Amy and me. After Amy's visit with Dr. Keel, we were instructed to stop by the lab on the ground floor of the physician building housing Dr. Keel's practice. The lab obtained blood from Amy, and we were told that the lab should have the test results back in about 48 hours at which time, Dr. Keel's office would call and inform us of the results.

Several days had passed without Amy and I hearing anything from Dr. Keel's office. We could not put off knowing any longer as to the answer of Amy being pregnant, and decided we would call to find out if they had an answer for us to confirm the positive results of Amy's home pregnancy test. Upon contacting Dr. Keel's office, Amy spoke with one of the doctor's staff members who placed her on hold to consult the office records. We were so happy to learn that they showed our results to be positive. We wasted no time to share this great news with family and close friends.

In our excitement, we wasted no time to go shop for baby clothes, a crib, bottles, and toys. In fact, in anticipation of the baby's birth we wasted no time to shop for the pending addition to our life. But soon after returning home from shopping, a message was left on our answering machine with a request to call Dr. Keel's office regarding Amy's pregnancy test results. Amy returned the call to the doctor's office and was told that her test results were inconclusive; she needed to make another trip to the laboratory to provide more blood samples. We were advised that Amy didn't need an appointment to have the additional lab samples taken and so we made it a priority to return as quickly as we could. This news thrust uncertainty back into a matter that we had already shared with people close to us.

How disappointing it was to learn that the doctor's office had reversed its prior confirmation. We were told the new lab results showed that Amy was not pregnant. In another conversation with Dr. Keel's office, we became aware that Amy was still on schedule to have the HSG test done in early December, made in a prior appointment with the doctor.

On December 6th, I arrived with Amy at the radiology clinic for the HSG, which was performed by Dr. Keel and lasted anywhere from 20 to 25 minutes. At the conclusion of the test, the doctor came out to discuss the findings with me and she explained that the hysterosalpingogram was quite uncomfortable for Amy, but they were able to complete the test. She said that the test showed there was no obstruction of flow, and this was good news. She did go on to say that she saw what appeared to be a cyst in the uterus and based on how it looked, the services of a specialist might be required – one that she already had in mind.

I was glad to hear that there was no medical abnormality or obstruction of fluid flow. This meant that Amy's reproductive organs were functioning properly. Of course, I always felt that Amy's ability to get pregnant was not an issue. There was just the question of whether she would be able to carry a child to term without miscarrying. At this time Amy only had the one miscarriage and being that it was quite an emotional drain on us, we didn't want to go through another miscarriage if at all possible. For us, the HSG was a diagnostic effort to minimize the risk of another miscarriage.

Dr. Keel and I agreed that the best route for Amy to take at this point was to see the recommended specialist. My reference for agreeing to this course of action was based on my knowledge that Amy's sister previously had a bout with cervical cancer and since this was in Amy's immediate family, hereditary genetics came into play. I didn't believe it was a stretch to assume the cyst that Dr. Keel said that she saw could be cancerous. I hoped and prayed that it wasn't, but I wanted to take no chances.

When Amy was brought back into the lobby from the back where they performed the HSG, she was quite upset about the level of discomfort caused by the procedure. She told me that this was something she would not go through again.

CHAPTER 3

December 13 (Three Months Before March 7)

Several days passed. The pre-dawn hours of December 13th brought snow with a decent accumulation so early in the winter for our location. The weather reports warned of snow flurries the days before, and my employer kept open the option to close the offices in the event of inclement weather. My instructions were to call and check my voicemail in the morning to see if I was required to come in. I got up pretty early that morning and looked outside the bedroom window. The air was cold, and I knew that I would see snow on the ground. I called in to retrieve my office voice messages and was glad to learn that I would have a day off due to snow.

When I hung up the phone after checking my voicemail message, I saw Amy walking to the bathroom. I was pretty concerned because she did get up several times throughout the night to go to the bathroom. This was not a common thing for her, but overnight there were many trips, in fact.

Through the bathroom door, I asked her if everything was okay. She told me that she had been bleeding since just before bedtime the prior evening, and that the bleeding was very heavy. Upon hearing this, I uncharacteristically picked up the phone and called Dr.

Keel's office. Amy always took the initiative to contact her doctor's office if she suspected something was wrong, but on this occasion I would be the one to make the call.

Since it was still pretty early in the day, I reached Dr. Keel's answering service, as they had not yet arrived at the office. I left a message for Dr. Keel that Amy was having frequent, heavy bleeding, and informed them that we would be waiting for a return call.

Eventually we received a call back from Dr. Keel's office. I answered and a woman identifying herself as being from Dr. Keel's office asked to speak with Amy. I gave Amy the phone and she began to explain what was happening. Amy hung up the phone and told me that they wanted her to go to the emergency room immediately.

We arrived at the University Hospital within an hour. The accumulation of overnight snow made driving a slow effort, not to mention the fact that our cold vehicle, which needed warming, was snow-covered and needed clearing off.

The distance from where we lived to that particular hospital is an 8-minute drive in normal conditions. When we got to the hospital, it didn't appear to be too busy. We stepped up immediately to check in, providing our information with me filling out the forms. Amy was provided a wheelchair and was taken into an examination room in the back.

A nurse examined Amy, asking her questions to confirm the accuracy of what was written on our completed paperwork. The nurse took Amy's vitals and explained to us that the doctor would be in to check on her. The attending physician was Dr. Bennett, an emergency staff doctor at University Hospital.

There were a number of medical things done to Amy that morning before Dr. Bennett came in to see her, but it didn't take long for him to realize what was happening. He had his chance to review the paperwork and test results before he gave us the news that Amy was in the process of miscarrying. Speechless, Amy and I just looked at each other for what felt like several minutes.

Probably sensing our surprise, Dr. Bennett broke our silence by asking us if we knew Amy was pregnant. Amy shook her head, and I told him that we didn't. I told the doctor that she couldn't possibly be pregnant because Amy's gynecologist couldn't confirm for us

16

that she was and in fact, told us that she wasn't. I explained to the doctor that Amy had taken a home pregnancy test approximately three to four weeks ago, and the home pregnancy test showed positive results. A subsequent visit with her gynecologist had determined that Amy was not pregnant, even though at first they told us that she was.

Dr. Bennett asked us if a urine test was done. Amy answered him, saying her doctor never requested a urine sample, only blood work.

Dr. Bennett asked us the name of the gynecologist and wanted to know the last time we saw "him". I replied that Amy's gynecologist was Dr. Keel, and the last time we saw "her" was almost a week ago when Amy had a procedure done at the specialty radiology clinic. He asked me about the procedure Amy underwent. I must have been in shock, because I couldn't remember the name of the test – neither could Amy. The only way I could tell him was to describe it.

"It's the test where they inject dye into the uterus and take x-rays," I said.

"An HSG?" he asked.

"Yes," I replied.

He abruptly looked at the nurse who was in the room with us. I couldn't see the nurse's expression because she was positioned behind us, but I didn't need to see either of them to know what they were thinking. If an HSG were done while Amy was actually pregnant, then that procedure contributed – if not caused – this current miscarriage.

Dr. Bennett said that Amy was going to need an emergency D&C and that he was going to call Dr. Keel. Before exiting the room, he whispered something to the nurse who was present; neither Amy or I could make out what he said to the nurse.

As Amy lay on the bed, she asked me why Dr. Keel couldn't verify her pregnancy. I don't remember answering her. I was seething, trying to answer the same question in my own mind. How in heaven's name could they miss confirming whether she was pregnant before performing the HSG? With anger churning in the pit of my stomach, it strangely began to give way to a feeling of gratitude. I realized how fortunate we were that I hadn't left for work and instead was available to bring her to the hospital. Since Amy doesn't drive well in the snow and with the nearest relatives living in a different quadrant of the metro, the fact that I was at home on this day when I'd normally have been at work was blessing, to say the least. Any other morning would have found me well on my way to work, which was about 22 miles from where we lived. I realized that the overnight snowfall helped me to be with my wife during this disappointing moment.

Amy wanted me to call her parents to inform them of her condition because they already knew she was at the hospital and was waiting for an update. Amy apparently called them before we left our apartment, when I was out cleaning snow off the car. I told Amy I would call them, but for the moment stepped out to take a walk through the hospital corridors instead. I really wasn't in the mood to talk right away and needed a moment to cool down, so I walked the halls for a few minutes to think.

I returned to the examination room where Amy was waiting, Dr. Bennett came back into the room not too long afterwards to inform Amy and I that he had spoke with Dr. Keel and that she was coming to the hospital to perform the emergency D&C. I nodded to convey that I understood and sat down beside Amy's bed to hold her hand.

Amy told me that while I was out, she reached her parents on the wireless phone and that they wanted me to call them after Dr. Keel arrived and performed her duties. The distance to the hospital and snow prevented my in-laws from making it to the hospital on this day, so they were dependent upon us to keep them informed.

The nurse came back in to inform us that Amy needed to be prepared for surgery before Dr. Keel's arrival and she asked us if Amy had anything to eat that morning. We were able to tell her that she had no meals since dinner of the night before. This was fortunate because of the general anesthesia Amy would need for the D&C.

After Amy and I talked, my anger started to subside. She didn't appear to be as upset as I was about things and I finally came to realize that since she was never convinced there even was a baby, it was somewhat easier to accept the loss. In other words, our hopes had already fallen when we were told by Dr. Keel's office that Amy wasn't pregnant. We didn't have time to get used to the idea that a baby was coming. It didn't stop the fact that there was hurt about the loss, but this was our way of putting the matter into perspective. Viewing it from this standpoint helped us to better cope with the loss.

Even after this, Amy never spoke ill of Dr. Keel. I began to understand that things like this must happen from time to time, and it's not necessarily the doctor's fault – not necessarily. My rational, forgiving side helped me to recognize that doctors are human, unperfect and entitled to an occasional professional mistake. Like any person, they can't be right 100% of the time. I thought through it logically and formed my own judgment about everything. I regarded this matter as a human error, and a significant professional failure.

They finished prepping Amy for the D&C, and she was wheeled off to an available room for the emergency procedure. The hospital staff directed me to the waiting area for patient family members. I figured this was a good time to call Amy's parents to inform them that their daughter was moments away from being worked on. Just as Amy's mother answered the phone and I was beginning to talk to her, Dr. Keel found me in the waiting room and walked over to me.

Quickly ending my conversation with my mother-in-law, I put the phone down on the receiver to speak with the doctor. I stood up to thank her for arriving so soon through the snow and cold weather. She dismissed my acknowledgement, saying that it was her intention to arrive as quickly as she could. She told me that since Amy was prepped and ready, she was going to go get started and would see me when everything was completed.

When the doctor left, I picked up the phone again to call Amy's parents. I spoke to her mother first, and then to her dad. In my conversation with Amy's Dad, I remember him asking me if the doctor made it to the hospital. When I responded that she had, he inquired if Amy and I ever considered changing physicians because to him it appeared that Dr. Keel didn't know what the hell she was doing. Then he commented on the doctor's inability to determine that Amy had been pregnant, and that in his opinion she didn't need to be practicing medicine if she couldn't confirm this most basic task expected of doctors in Dr. Keel's specialty. My father-in-law tends to shoot from the hip. He's quite straightforward, non-mincing with his words. I partially agreed with his summary of things but told him I was reluctant to change doctors because Amy and I had been seeing Dr. Keel from the very beginning. We were familiar with her, and she was familiar with us, and that the idea of having to find a new doctor to familiarize ourselves with while trying to get the new doctor up to speed on Amy's medical history wasn't something we were necessarily willing to go through.

The D&C procedure lasted nearly an hour, judging from the time I last saw Dr. Keel to the time I saw her again. Again, Dr. Keel found me in the waiting room again and came over to sit down beside me.

"Everything went well," Dr. Keel said. After a few seconds of silence she then began to apologize, saying that she was very sorry that her office wasn't able to verify Amy's pregnancy. Dr. Keel admitted that if she had verified Amy's pregnancy, she would never have performed the HSG. She said that Amy's hormone readings were low, and this prevented her from determining whether Amy was pregnant. Then she suggested that perhaps Amy wasn't really pregnant, but instead possibly had residual placental tissue left from the first D&C she performed several months earlier. Perhaps she said this as an effort to diminish liability, because she didn't seem confident when she offered this theory. In fact, she appeared quite baffled when she even offered it as a suggestion. Dr. Bennett, the attending ER physician, was much more convincing in his diagnosis that Amy had miscarried, and so I was more inclined to believe what he already told me.

Continuing my conversation with Dr. Keel in the hospital lobby, I asked her if it were likely that the cyst she believed she had seen from the HSG test was really a fertilized egg attached to the uterine wall. She replied that this was a possible assumption. I then asked her that if this were true, would it be necessary for Amy to begin seeing the specialist we had discussed in the lobby after the HSG test. Dr. Keel thought for a moment before replying, telling me that it wouldn't be necessary for Amy to start seeing the specialist we talked about on December 6th.

Dr. Keel asked if we had our next appointment scheduled with her office. I responded that the appointment was already set sometime in January, the next month. Dr. Keel said that she would go over some obstetric options with us during our next visit, and then told me that Amy was being moved to recovery and that a nurse would come get me when I was able to see her. After Dr. Keel performed this second D&C, it never entered my mind to inquire or press this incident any further because as far as Amy and I were concerned it was simply a clinical mistake – I suppose. Because we seemed to have a rapport with Dr. Keel, we didn't consider changing physicians. In fact, Amy and I would come to discuss the HSG/miscarriage situation days later and opted to retain our trust in Dr. Keel's ability.

It was only a few minutes before a nurse found me in the waiting room to take me to where Amy was. I followed the nurse back into the recovery room. When I saw Amy she was lying on her back, obviously groggy from the general anesthesia from the procedure. She had tears falling vertically from both eyes down to her ears. She moaned as the nurses talked to her to get her coherent enough to drink some water and eat crackers. She would be able to leave once she was awake enough to get dressed.

At discharge, we were given prescriptions to have filled with instructions to follow for the next couple of days. By the time we left the hospital it was late in the afternoon. I took Amy home so that she could rest while I went to have her prescriptions filled. After doing so I returned home and catered her needs so that she could stay off her feet. We remained in each other's company for the rest of that cold, wet, snowy day.

From this moment on Dr. Keel would regard this incident as "residual placental and fetal tissue". She had concluded that the first D&C she performed on Amy did not result in complete removal of the fetal tissue and had made this second emergency D&C necessary which contradicted Dr. Bennett's diagnosis altogether. It is more likely that the HSG directly contributed to the second miscarriage.

CHAPTER 4

Day 1: March 7 – 6:22 AM

The day arrived when I was to take my wife to the Northwest Presbyterian Medical Center for the scheduled outpatient surgery recommended to us by Dr. Keel. It was the middle of the week. The local time was just before 6:30 in the morning and because Amy and I underestimated the time we had to get to the hospital, we were running slightly behind.

There was really nothing different about this day than any of the other times Amy went to a medical appointment. Both of us had taken the day off from our respective jobs for the purpose of Amy having this same-day surgery. My intention was to return to work the following day, assuming Amy's surgery went okay and there were no special instructions to have her observed a day after discharge.

Although the operation was scheduled for 10:00 a.m., our instructions were to arrive by 6:30 in the morning for check-in, paperwork, and prepping purposes. We were quite unsure exactly where we needed to go after we arrived at the hospital, and realizing the time was right on the button, we ran through the parking lot to the hospital entrance. Once we were inside the hospital, it did not take long for us to find the receptionist to get our information from her.

The receptionist located Amy's name on the list and gave us instructions on where we needed to go from there. We followed the receptionist's instructions and found ourselves at the day-surgery nurse's station where we were greeted and asked to fill out paperwork. The hospital's standard pre-op paperwork included a *Conditions of Treatment and Admission* form, a form on *Patient Rights and Responsibilities*, information regarding *Advanced Directive* and *Consent for Treatment*. These forms accompanied the other forms that we had to fill out relating to our insurance and personal information.

After completing the paperwork, Amy was asked to undress and put on one of those infamous hospital gowns – the ones that expose the backside if not carefully tied. We were given a plastic bag in which to place her clothing and other personal belongings, which I held onto from this moment on.

Amy was asked to step onto a scale on the other side of the room. She weighed in at her normal weight, which was anywhere between 108 to 112 pounds. A hospital patient identification tag was placed on her wrist, and we talked with the hospital's admitting clerk about the paperwork that we had completed just moments earlier. The clerk verified all the information written on the forms by asking Amy a few questions. She then made a phone call to another area of the hospital to inform them that Amy's check-in paperwork was complete.

A nurse came in to get us and take us to the day surgery prepping rooms on the same floor. The place where we were taken was a big room which had drapes dividing it into smaller sections, each section containing a bed. We followed the nurse into one of the sections, and the nurse assisted Amy onto a bed and began to rub iodine on her arm for placement of the IV. As she worked, the nurse asked Amy some of the same questions the clerk did earlier, just to make sure that Amy had followed the preoperative instructions regarding food intake and such.

When she completed the insertion of the IV, the nurse asked Amy if there was anything she needed. Amy asked for an extra pillow and more sheets to cover up. The air in the hospital was almost too cool to be comfortable. The nurse left and returned with the pillow and extra sheets. The nurse reminded us that Amy's surgery was scheduled for 10:00, and that we would have to wait for the anesthesiologist and Dr. Keel. I looked at my watch and realized that it wasn't yet passed 8:00 a.m.

It would be a long wait before the doctors came to get her, so Amy and I filled up the time with conversation. We used the back of our patient copy form to write on. We played several games of tic-tac-toe, and soon became bored with it. Amy used the remaining area of the page to doodle. She drew a picture of a woman's face and then wrote down how she was feeling. I read what she had written: "I wish they would hurry up – I am so sleepy." Seeing this, I laughed because this was exactly how I was feeling. I held her hand as we waited for them to come and get her.

It wasn't hard for me to understand that Amy was exhausted. She worked a nine-hour shift the night before and didn't get off until 11:30 p.m. By the time she made it home, she only had about 4½ to 5 hours of sleep before getting to the hospital the next morning.

Amy worked in retail and that job had weird hours. The position she held before this was that of a CNA at a local nursing home. After being a CNA for several years she appreciated the vocational change that retail provided. She didn't want to return to the nursing home arena if she could avoid it. Her desire to drop the CNA profession was due to the long weekend hours, low pay, and constant staffing issues. She also complained about how difficult it was when certain residents died after she allowed herself to become close to them.

Being a former CNA was just one of the reasons Amy wasn't a stranger to medical settings. Obviously, her prior doctor's office appointments and outpatient procedures made her accustomed to the setting she found herself on this day. Understandably she wasn't too happy about being at the hospital on this particular day, and said she was anxious for the surgery to be over. I agreed. The path that brought us to this point was never anticipated, but Amy's doctor seemed to feel this would resolve her obstetric matters. Amy and I both hoped that this procedure would produce results to help us get on with our lives.

The surgical procedure that Amy was to undergo was a hysteroscopy and laparoscopy.

A hysteroscopy is a diagnostic surgical procedure that allows examination inside the uterus without an incision into the abdominal wall. A lighted instrument called a hysteroscope is inserted through the pelvis and into the uterus, transmitting images of the uterus from the inside onto a screen. If it were determined that there was indeed a uterine septum, then the tissue could be removed during the hysteroscopy with the laparoscope, since it is common for other instruments to be used along with the hysteroscope for treatment. This hysteroscopy was to be performed in conjunction with laparoscopy.

A laparoscopy is a surgical procedure used to examine abdominal or female pelvic organs. During a laparoscopy, a small incision is made in the abdomen and a thin, lighted tube called a laparoscope is inserted into the abdomen. It is usual for a hysteroscopy or laparoscopy to be performed as separate procedures on a patient, but not uncommon to have them both performed simultaneously, as would happen on this day in Amy's situation.

At our consultation visit with Dr. Keel in January, regarding the hysteroscopy/laparoscopy procedure, the doctor stressed the need for Amy to have this surgery. There were no alternative options discussed. The doctor was confident that this procedure would eliminate the uterine septum that questionably caused Amy to first miscarry in the summer, prior to our consultation visit with Dr. Keel in January. Dr. Keel explained to us that the laparoscopy was necessary so that during the hysteroscopy, the uterus could be viewed from the topside to allow greater visibility when removing the septum tissue. This would eliminate a "blind effort" at trying to remove the septum. During this appointment, we were also advised that there were certain unspecific risks, but without going into any detail the doctor assured us that she had performed this procedure many times without ever encountering any of the risks. Amy and I were at ease knowing that the doctor was experienced in performing the procedure absent of any complications. The entire consultation was rather brief and to-the-point, lasting only three or four minutes.

Of course, our hopes rested on the successful completion of the surgery. It would give us the opportunity to stop having recurring appointments at the doctor's office and start moving ahead with our lives. If it were meant for us to have children, then perhaps the hysteroscopy/laparoscopy procedure would be the answer for moving us a step closer to that possibility.

CHAPTER 5

10:04 AM

This early day in March appeared to be a busy one for the hospital. There were probably 20 people or more in the waiting room. I was glad that in spite of the number of people present, there were a number of open chairs available. I wanted to find a seat that was near a table with magazines and isolated from the other folks in the room. I wasn't particularly interested in having a conversation with anyone, so I found a location where few others were. After locating my spot and sitting down, I picked up a magazine and buried my attention in it.

After a while I looked at my watch and noticed it had been a little over an hour since Amy was taken into surgery. I was expecting to be informed soon of the surgery's completion. 45 minutes was my benchmark, as this was the approximate time I was given for the length of the surgery. When it passed, I really didn't think much of it because I had an understanding that delays are often common in matters medically related.

As I sat in the waiting room browsing through a magazine, I heard an overhead page that said: "Vascular surgeon to operating room four, stat - we need a vascular surgeon to operating room four, stat!" Being a former employee at a hospital, I understood that it wasn't uncommon to hear such a request over the intercom, and I really didn't think much more about it. I continued looking through the magazine in my hands. Roughly five minutes later, a second page like the first was announced overhead: "We need a vascular surgeon to operating room four, stat - any available vascular surgeon to operating room four, stat!"

I remember thinking to myself that 5 minutes was a long time between pages for the same emergency request. I hoped that the person for whom this call was announced was getting good care. The page could have been for any patient's relative in the waiting room, as there were still several people occupying the waiting room.

A few seconds after the second page, the phone rang in the waiting room. There was an elderly woman dressed in a pink and white candy-striped shirt manning the receptionist station in the middle of the room. This volunteer answered the phone and then called into the room, asking for a Mr. Larren. Standing to my feet I made my way over to the desk and told the woman who I was. She gave me the phone stating that the call was for me. On the other end of this call was a hospital staff member who said that she was calling on behalf of the operating room where Amy was being treated. This voice on the phone said that there was a slight development in Amy's procedure that I needed to be aware of and that Dr. Keel would come out to explain details to me. She told me that Amy was doing okay and reaffirmed that Dr. Keel would be out to talk more with me. Initially, I didn't really know what to make of this call and ultimately just took it for what it was: an announcement of pending information to come.

I went back to my seat and sat down. I hardly returned to my magazine when I noticed two nurses speaking with the volunteer at the desk, the one who had answered the phone. The volunteer pointed in my direction and the nurses walked over to where I was seated. One of them said my name and I stood up to greet them. They asked me to have a seat and the two of them sat down in the adjacent seats on my left that were positioned against the wall perpendicular to mine. One of them began, "Mr. Larren, we were sent in to advise you that there was a slight complication with Amy in the operating room. She is doing well and being handled with the best of care, but we wanted to let you know that the doctor will be out to talk with you about it very soon."

Since they reported that Amy was doing well despite the development, I had no doubts that she was in good hands and asked them if the doctor was successful in removing the uterine septum. The two nurses looked at each other before replying to my question. The second nurse said she didn't know about the details of the surgery and confessed they were not in the operating room where Amy was being worked on. It puzzled me that they were sent to give me the information about my wife but didn't have any real information to convey, other than news about the slight complication. Understanding that they had no additional information to give me, I immediately wondered if the page requests for a vascular surgeon I had heard just moments earlier were related to my wife.

"Is Amy in operating room four? Is Dr. Keel still with her?" I asked. They affirmed that Amy's surgery was being performed in operating room four, and as far as they knew Dr. Keel was still with her. They told me that the doctor should be out to talk with me in about ten minutes. With nothing else to ask, I thanked them for coming to tell me about the development. They got up and departed the waiting room.

As the nurses walked away from me, I wondered what the doctor would tell me and what questions I would ask her after she came in. I glanced at all the people in the room, wondering what their doctors would have to tell them about the loved ones they were here to support. I further thought about how many of these people had loved ones who would be returning home this afternoon and how many would have to stay the night at the hospital.

Some time had passed and again I glanced at my wristwatch, noticing it was well past the ten minutes since the nurses departed. They told me that Dr. Keel would be out to talk with me in about ten minutes, and since it was nearly an hour since I spoke to anyone regarding Amy's care, I became more agitated with every minute that passed without me seeing the doctor.

Dr. Keel finally arrived in the waiting room. She approached me and sat down in the seat across from mine. She greeted me without any conspicuous change in her attitude or tone and began re-explaining the procedure that Amy came in for and added that after the incision was made she saw blood as she was maneuvering the scope to the site. She commented that the blood indicated that there was internal bleeding. Not wanting to miss why she was seeing blood, she said she had to remove the scope and open Amy's abdomen to determine exactly where the blood was coming from and to stop it. She told me that because of the blood loss, Amy needed a transfusion. She said that Amy was currently in great shape but that her surgery was no longer outpatient. Amy would have to remain overnight in the hospital as inpatient.

Dr. Keel asked me if I had any questions. I asked her if she knew why she had seen blood once she started the procedure, she replied that the trocar, the penetrating instrument used to make an incision through the abdominal wall, has a plastic spring-loaded protective sheath. It apparently malfunctioned during the procedure and was suspect to the reason she saw blood after entry into the abdominal wall. She told me that they had to open Amy's abdomen to locate the hemorrhaging and stop it.

I then asked her the same question I had earlier asked the two nurses. I wanted to know if the septum had been removed. Dr. Keel told me that she was able to determine that there was indeed a septum, but the surgical procedure did not progress to the point where it was removed. I assumed that the injury prevented her from completing the procedure.

Before her departure, Dr. Keel told me that Amy had the best doctors working on her, that she was returning to the OR where Amy was and that they would be moving Amy into recovery in another 20 to 30 minutes. She said I would be notified once Amy was ready to be moved. After she departed, I sat there and thought for a moment. I was concerned that the surgery for removal of the uterine septum was a failure and the fact that, medically speaking, we were still in the same boat that we were in before we arrived. I would come to learn that Amy and I would have been very fortunate *if* this were true.

Still in the waiting room, I became bored with the magazine and began to watch the TV monitor mounted on the wall across the room. It felt as if I had been sitting there for a very long time. Roughly 80 - 90 minutes would pass before I would hear anything from the OR. I was so tired and wanted to recline to sleep, but this wasn't the time or place to rest.

The phone rang and I reactively looked over to the desk to see if it were for me. I finally received another phone call. I got up and went over to the desk to take the call. Someone calling from the operating room told me that Amy was still in surgery and that if I was waiting to eat lunch, then now would probably be a good time to go. I thought this was a good idea and was glad that they called to let me know. It was after 1:00 in the afternoon and I was feeling a bit hungry.

I told the volunteer at the desk that I was going to go have lunch and she smiled as she acknowledged my message.

Since I didn't have any cash with me at all, I stepped onto the elevator and descended to the ground floor to exit the building. Our apartment was about ten minutes away from the hospital and I decided that I would go home and have a TV dinner for lunch rather than use the hospital's ATM to spend money I knew I might need for upcoming medical bills.

The weather outside was clear, bright, and sunny. By this time, it was between 1:15 and 1:30 in the afternoon. The lunch rush hour traffic usually subsides at 2:00, and since the lunch rush hour traffic was still prevalent, it added time to my usually 10-minute commute to our apartment. I figured as long as I was back at the hospital within an hour then I wouldn't be missed.

When I got to the apartment, I called my parents who live about 75 miles outside of our local area. They were aware that Amy was having surgery today and wanted me to communicate with them when everything was finished, just to let them know that things were fine. I dialed the number to my parents' house.

My dad answered the phone. As I began talking to him, I took a TV dinner out of the icebox and began opening it to place into the microwave. I informed Dad about the events that had happened so far, and he obviously wanted to know more about Amy's condition. I told him as far as I knew she was doing well, adding that Amy would be staying in the hospital rather than coming home that afternoon as originally planned. He wanted me to keep him posted on everything that was happening, and then put my mom on the phone so I could tell her the information I had just shared with him. I quickly brought Mom up to speed about the situation and she conveyed to me her uneasiness of this news and told me to be sure to keep her abreast of Amy's situation.

I had nearly completed my conversation with Mom when an incoming phone call prompted me to end my talk with my mother. I switched over to answer the incoming call and was surprised that it was my mother-in-law, Helen.

Now speaking with my mother-in-law, she inquired why I was not at the hospital with Amy. I replied, telling her that I had just came home to eat lunch, which the operating room advised me that I could because Amy was still in surgery. My mother-in-law then told me that Dr. Keel's office had just called her house trying to locate me. Helen added that the call sounded urgent, but they would not give her any specific information. She told me that I needed to get back to the hospital ASAP and to call her as soon as I could so that she could know how Amy was doing. I told her I was returning to the hospital right away and I would call her back as soon as I found out what was going on. I cancelled the microwave before it finished cooking my box meal. It was obvious that lunch was going to have to wait.

Only seconds after ending my conversation with my mother-in-law, my phone rang again just as I was stepping out the door. "Hello?" I answered. It was an employee from Dr. Keel's office telling me that she was calling on behalf of Dr. Keel and that I needed to return to the hospital. When I tried to get information from this woman who was on the phone, she said that she had no information to tell me other than the fact that I needed to get back to the Presbyterian Medical Center.

I quickly rushed out of the apartment and ran to the car. My drive back to the hospital from the apartment did not seem to take as long as my drive from the hospital. It was the route and the same distance, but the circumstances motivating each trip were quite different.

CHAPTER 6

1:47 PM

I pulled my car into the first available parking space upon my arrival at the hospital. While walking briskly to the hospital entrance, I couldn't remember if I had locked the door to the apartment before rushing off. But it was too late to be concerned about that now. I made it back to the hospital and the news inside was of greater importance.

After entering the facility, I was well into the hospital when I spotted Dr. Keel running towards me. I don't know if the fact that I encountered her here was by design or by accident, but we met in the hallway just a few feet short of me reaching the elevators.

When I looked at Dr. Keel, I could see that her demeanor had changed, and she appeared quite frantic. The worry on her face was not easily hidden. Call me naïve, but for the first time in all the day's events I suddenly realized that something was terribly wrong. Upon this realization came my suspicion that Amy's condition was far worse than Dr. Keel or the hospital staff had initially let on.

Dr. Keel looked at me and told me that she had been trying to reach me. I replied to her that per the operating room's recommendation, I went to have lunch. I asked her to tell me what was going on and she answered, saying Amy had to be taken back into surgery. She reminded me again that Amy was given a transfusion and told me that Amy remained stable for some time. She continued, saying that she left the OR while the other medical members worked on Amy. When she returned to check on Amy, she discovered that Amy's vitals had declined significantly, and that emergent surgical intervention was necessary. The information as it was unveiled was pretty sketchy, but I resisted inquiring specifics because I wanted the doctor's full attention back on Amy.

I was distraught by the fact that my wife was not doing well and told Dr. Keel that I wanted to be kept abreast of *everything* going on with Amy. She asked me where she would be able to reach me, to which I replied that I would be in the surgery waiting room and that I would not be going *anywhere*.

Immediately, I returned to the waiting room, and I knew I had to call my mother-in-law, Helen, to update her on Amy's condition. I used the hospital's phone in the waiting room to call and when she answered I could hear the fear in her voice. It may have been a mother's intuition that caused Helen to be quicker than I at recognizing the fact that Amy was in dire shape, and she told me in no uncertain terms that she was on her way to the hospital.

After talking with Amy's mom, I called my supervisor at work to explain the situation. I advised him that I was shifting my priority solely upon my wife and to not expect me at work until further notice. If he had any objection to what I had just told him, he wasn't going to be so bold as to tell me during *this* conversation.

When my phone call ended, I could feel the eyes of people in the waiting room staring at me. I guess they knew that my situation was a bad one since I had received several phone calls in the waiting room and the fact that I had spoken to the nurses and Dr. Keel in this same area earlier in the day.

I don't know what expression was on my face but as the strangers watched me, I slowly made my way to a chair in the corner. I sat down and stared unfocused at the floor. The room felt like it was spinning, and I felt nauseous.

It wasn't long before a professionally dressed woman entered the waiting room and asked the candy striper volunteer sitting at the desk where I could be found. This much I gathered based on the volunteer's action of lifting a hand and pointing at me. The professionally dressed lady made her way to where I was, and she introduced herself as the Administrator of the Northwest Presbyterian Medical Center. I looked at the nametag on her black jacket to verify her introduction.

I don't recall the entirety of my conversation with this woman, but I do remember asking her specific questions about my wife's condition. Without giving me much additional information, she apologized to me about my situation and she assured me that the physicians and hospital staff would do everything they possibly could for Amy. She told me that Dr. Keel would come out to update me soon and volunteered to send up snacks for me and any other family members that might be arriving. Then she asked me if I would object to speaking with a chaplain.

I really didn't know how to take her question. Had she asked me this because she knew more than she was telling me? Or, did she ask me this out of respect of my Christian faith? One of the questions on the pre-op paperwork that we filled in during admittance was a question about our religion. I remember watching Amy as she filled in the answer, *Southern Baptist*, on the questionnaire.

I couldn't make myself ask the Administrator why she asked me this. Perhaps I knew she wouldn't give me any additional info, or maybe I was just afraid to know the true answer if she did. It was possible the chaplain may be more forthcoming with the answers I wasn't getting from the Hospital Administrator. But even if I couldn't get additional information from the chaplain, I understood there was never a bad time to pray, so I told the Administrator that I would accept speaking with a chaplain.

The Hospital Administrator ushered me into a private waiting room away from everybody else, just around the corner from the main waiting area. She asked me to have a seat and that the chaplain would be with me momentarily. She exited the room and closed the door behind her.

I thought it odd that the chaplain arrived as quickly as he did because when he entered the room I wasn't as ready to talk with him as I initially thought. As I stood to greet him, we shook hands and the gentleman introduced himself to me as Collin. We sat down and he asked me how he could help.

I asked Collin if he could tell me what he knew about my wife. He replied that he didn't know anything about our situation or why we were here, other than the fact that the Administrator informed him that Amy had arrived for surgery and now was receiving emergency care. He asked me what Amy had come in for and as I tried to explain to him why she was here, a cold chill gripped me.

I grasped the fact that I really didn't know anything. I hadn't seen her since they wheeled her off to surgery just before 10:00 in the morning, and it was already in the middle of the afternoon. We continued to talk a little more – I don't remember any details of that conversation other than it was brief – and he listened more than he spoke. He finally asked me if I would object to him praying with me. I had no objection to praying and told him so. We bowed our heads and Collin led the prayer.

It wasn't long after praying that two of Amy's friends, Karyn and Karla, entered the private waiting room where the chaplain and I were. Introductions were made. The chaplain didn't leave right away but soon after he did, Heather, Amy's younger sister, appeared, and then my mother-in-law, Helen, arrived. Upon Helen's arrival, I filled them all in on what I knew at this point and told her that I was waiting for Dr. Keel to come in and update me further.

A short while after the arrival of Amy's sister and mother, a complimentary food tray was delivered to the room, fulfilling the Hospital Administrator's offer to provide snacks. The round tray was about two feet in diameter, filled with vegetables, fruit, packaged snacks, and iced cans of beverages and bottled water were furnished in a separate large container. It was rather apparent that the hospital intended this as a gesture of amends and sympathy for the family. Although impressive, seeing this huge tray of refreshments did little to ease my concern, and at this moment I felt that I needed to detach myself from the others in the room. The chill that had gripped me before everyone's arrival just wouldn't subside.

Because of my realization that not every victim of medical negligence survives, I have given much weight and consideration of whether to include the next few paragraphs in this book. Some may question or doubt the implication of divine intervention. If this is you, then feel free to skip on to the next chapter. However, my decision to include this private moment is based on events I experienced, from my perspective and my sincere belief that the outcome would have been gravely different had I not considered the course and acted. This part of our experience is a key component of the whole and I determined that omitting it would be a reckless failure to convey our whole story in the most truthful manner.

In deep despair, there was little doubt over what I had to do next. It's one thing to be led in prayer by a chaplain, and something more urgently profound to personally initiate prayer independently. As a Christian, I knew I had the potency of prayer, and I took some comfort in knowing nothing here was happening without God's own knowledge of the situation. I realized that Amy's health as well as the whole situation was totally out of my hands. I left the private waiting room and went to the single restroom back in the main waiting area. I locked the door. I could feel the perspiration underneath my clothing and found my face wet with tears. Clasping my hands together I bowed my head at the sink and sank to my knees. It would be the most intense prayer moment that I had ever experienced up to that time.

My prayer began with a confession of personal sins – which is not formulary, but rather, necessary, to clear darkness from my heart. Amy was object of my prayer, but the focus behind my prayer was the knowledge and belief that God was powerful enough to intervene. It was my unwavering belief in God and *His* ability that compelled me to pray. Nothing puts one in the mode to seek God than helplessness. Honestly, I couldn't have been more helpless.

I remember appealing to God that He owed me nothing and that He had every right to deny my request. I told God that if He never did another thing for me, He would have already done enough for me. I remember telling Him that I wish I could somehow take Amy's place and asked for His will to be that Amy survived this predicament. I prayed that the doctors treating her would put their best skills forward and asked for His guidance for me to know how to handle these critical moments.

The component that made this prayer so intense was not just the fact that I felt God's presence – it was the concentrated, undistracted focus of my belief in God's ability. There was the reality that Christ allowed sinners like me to beckon the mercy of God, and it's only through Christ that this is possible. Never had this promise been so evident to me than at that very moment.

God answers prayer differently to different people. I knew that non-Christians didn't have the power of prayer available to them unless a Christian prayed on their behalf. I'm no theologian, but I knew that there were certain promises God gave to His children that others cannot claim, and as an admitted child of God I made my appeal to him – not out of selfishness – but out of gratitude.

In the many days before the surgery, Amy and I had been serving God through our regular attendance at church and in regular bible study. My personal growth towards God was a relationship that had been cultivated since my mid-teen years. This knowledge of God was found only through my belief and knowledge of Christ, and despite what the non-Christian world may claim, knowing Jesus Christ is the *only* way to know God. My marriage to Amy allowed our growth in our Christian faith to become another facet of our growth to each other. This is paramount because many people believe that they have the right to summon the attention of God in a helpless situation, expecting His attention without ever cultivating a personal relationship with Him in everyday life prior to a crisis. Amy and I were faithful servants to the teachings of Christ and regularly attended church. As a result, I knew God would hear me, even if I didn't know that He would respond in the way that I wanted.

It's tough to accurately describe my frame of mind at that moment in time other than to say I had confidence that even if Amy did not survive, things would somehow be okay. I knew in whom my hope was, and this became a great source of strength. I was still very scared that I might lose her, but there was an underlying confidence that God's will — whatever it was — would prevail.

After praying, I looked in the mirror and saw bloodshot eyes staring back at me. It was here that I realized that prayer was going to be the key if Amy were to survive. I determined that my next course of action would be to enlist the prayers of other Christians by getting Amy on a prayer chain. While everything else was out of my hands, I determined this was the *one* thing I could do on her behalf. In this sense, I wasn't quite as helpless as I had originally thought and had a sense of purpose from this point forward.

Remarkably, it was during this very week that a statewide pastor's conference was taking place locally. My sister, Robyn, along with her husband, Chris, was in our city attending the conference. Chris was the pastor of a church in the city of their residence, which was the same community where my parents lived. This same brother-in-law had performed Amy's and my wedding ceremony less than a year earlier. He and my sister had some knowledge of Amy's medical events leading up to the scheduled outpatient surgery Amy was having that day and wanted to know when she was released post-surgery. But they did not know all the complications that had happened that morning. I had their mobile number, and I felt compelled to call and update them on the situation at hand — the best I could.

Before unlocking and opening the restroom door, I tried my best to hide my emotional evidence by washing off my face in cold water and putting contact lens rewetting drops in my eyes. The rewetting drops were something I always carried in my pocket, especially during the spring months to combat the dryness often accompanied with wearing contact lenses, plus the allergens the season brought to this part of the country. The droplets did little to remove any of the redness of my eyes. Despite this, I knew I had to get back to the waiting room so that I wouldn't miss the doctor's update.

I unlocked and opened the bathroom door, then moved to an inconspicuous, unpopulated area of the hospital to call my brother-in-law. I had no trouble reaching him and I updated him of everything that had occurred. He was disturbed by my news. I asked him to place Amy on every prayer list he could find. He assured me they would do their part to get her placed on prayer lists. At the time that I called, he and my sister were in a restaurant having dinner with some of their clergy friends, and he took the moment to share Amy's situation with those present at the table. I would come to learn (months later) that they immediately prayed for Amy right at the table where they were having dinner.

Over the next few days, I would notify as many people as I could to contact as many people as they could to get Amy added on prayer lists. Imagine having a team of Christian saints praying corporately for the same cause. I would come to discover that – through personal contacts of my friends and their friends – Amy would be on prayer lists in as many as five states!

CHAPTER 7

5:43 PM

After my phone call to my brother-in-law, I returned to the waiting room where the family members gathered and noticed that a few others had arrived. Amy's older sister, Crystal, and her husband, Derek, were there. Gail, a close friend of Amy's mother, had also arrived. I explained to all present what I could about everything that I knew up to that point. Naturally, there were many questions and very few answers. We were all anticipating the arrival of Dr. Keel to explain Amy's injury, update us on her condition, and answer some of the questions that we needed answering.

Eventually, Dr. Keel entered the waiting room accompanied by another medical staff member – possibly her nurse. Amy's mother was identified to Dr. Keel by someone in the room. Dr. Keel sat down and proceeded to explain events leading up to Amy's injuries. The details were told to Amy's mother in a very similar fashion as they were told to me, still somewhat vague. There was no admission of personal guilt or error by Dr. Keel and she again made mention of the defective scalpel device that was suspect to the reason Amy was injured during surgery. The doctor in her explanation seemed to describe Amy's injury as if it were *detected* during the procedure as opposed to being caused by it.

39

Dr. Keel ended her explanation of Amy's injury by trying to put a positive spin on the situation, commenting that Amy was in the best place to recover from her type of injuries since the hospital had on hand all the necessary equipment and personnel available to deal with this type of emergency. She said we were fortunate that Amy was at the Northwest Presbyterian Medical Center than at any other hospital in the metro. This didn't make me feel any better about the situation and aside from what was already said, Dr. Keel *could not* assure us that Amy would make it through this.

Amy's mother asked several questions of Dr. Keel, but there was really no revelation of additional information that we hadn't already heard. When Dr. Keel finished answering Helen's questions, she informed us that Dr. Ferris, one of the surgeons who worked on Amy, would be in to update us before Amy was transported from recovery. After Dr. Keel left there was a deafening silence in the room and for me a dismal feeling of confusion and disbelief.

The silence was broken when those present in the waiting room began discussing Amy's injuries. As we understood things, it appeared to us that Amy's initial injury was that of a nick, tear or severing of a major blood vessel – perhaps the vena cava – in her abdomen, which resulted in heavy blood loss. This would later be confirmed, but the lingering question we couldn't quite figure out was how the second injury regarding the central line blood transfusion happened and how much damage this caused.

Dr. Ferris finally made it into the private waiting room where we were all sitting. He was rather young-looking for someone with his said skill. He was dressed in scrubs and wore glasses. I was introduced to Dr. Ferris as Amy's husband. I stood to shake his hand and as he looked me straight in the eye, he was slow to begin speaking. He summarized Amy's condition, saying that because she lost a lot of blood she had to have a transfusion to replace that which was lost. Sometime after the transfusion it was discovered that she began to have a sharp drop in blood pressure, and she had to be rushed back into surgery to perform an emergency procedure – an operation on the thorax or upper chest area – to correct the problem. This emergency operation was a thoracotomy. Somehow the blood that Amy had received from the transfusion missed entering her blood stream and filled her chest cavity, essentially drowning her in addition to denying her blood and oxygen to vital organs.

Dr. Ferris continued, saying that they obviously had many concerns. He said that their primary concern was that of organ failure; beginning foremost with the kidneys, then eventually other organs, system failure, and the possibility that she could very well die. He told me that even if Amy were to survive, complications expected due to the lack of blood circulation would likely have resulted in brain damage, leaving her in a vegetative state. He stated that, as surgeons, they had done all that they could do and at this point she just had to be monitored closely. He added that the first 24 hours were always the most critical. What Amy had going for her was her youth. He shared all of this with me in the most tactful way. I nodded my head, acknowledging everything he had just told me. For fear of breaking down, I had no questions to ask him.

After the meeting with Dr. Ferris, I found myself thinking the unthinkable. I kept asking myself how in the universe we got here. An otherwise healthy young woman that had come in for a rather routine outpatient surgery was now on the threshold of death, fighting for her life. To me, this situation was unforeseeable and with each passing minute and with every encounter with a doctor or hospital staff member, I felt more and more as if the situation was deteriorating. I had not discounted my prayer from earlier, but I was just taken aback at how quickly things could get so terribly complicated and life-threatening.

I always knew that with *any* surgery there were certain risks that came into play, but I also knew that during surgery, Amy would be in a controlled environment with many "controllables" in place to minimize risks. This was a scheduled procedure, one that the doctor admitted she had performed many times without incident and this fact gave me a sense of security, which turned out to be false. It was hard for me to fathom how things became so dire in this surgery, especially since it appeared that there was not one, but *two* errors made, the second one substantially complicating matters for Amy.

The fact that I had not seen Amy for several hours tore at my conscious. I had no way of knowing if I would ever see her again the way she was that morning before the surgery. What if she had already flat-lined and these people were just attempting to lower my expectations that she might recover before telling me that she had passed? The negative thoughts kept coming and the temptation to give up hope was nearly overwhelming. Yet, I determined that if I could just see her, I would be able to hold onto the hope that the prayers on our behalf would impact the outcome.

41

When Dr. Ferris left the room, one of Amy's friends began crying, saying that the lower portion of the doctor's scrubs were very bloody from below the knees. I did not notice this when I talked with Dr. Ferris, but those who saw it assumed that he had just come from working on Amy and the blood was a tell-tell sign of the magnitude of the trauma.

The atmosphere in the room was suddenly very solemn.

CHAPTER 8

6:02 PM

Medial staff personnel were quite aware of my desire to see my wife. Earlier I was told that the hospital had a policy against allowing family members to see the patient before being removed from the recovery area. Based on the circumstances, the hospital wisely annulled the policy and allowed me to see Amy while she was in recovery, prior to her being moved to the ICU. They allowed me to choose one other person to come with me; there was no question that Amy's mother would accompany me to the recovery room.

When the time came to go see Amy, Helen and I left the private waiting room and followed a nurse around the corner and down a hall. We passed through some double doors, and we had reached our destination: a cold room with drapes dividing the bed positions. Amy was in the first position and there were three medical staff workers hovering over her. When the workers moved out of the way, neither Helen nor I were prepared for what we saw.

I froze as I looked her over, and Amy's mother gasped while placing her hands over her mouth, as if trying to hold in her emotions. My once beautiful wife lay there on the bed in a terrifying picture of brutal injury. She was not the same person I brought into the hospital that same morning.

43

Seeing her, the first thing I noticed were the many tubes and IV lines running all over her body, to and from these machines and monitors placed near the bed. She was covered in blood and as I forced myself closer, I could see wet blood on the side of her neck. The blood was in her ears, in her mouth, on her teeth and saturated in her hair. There appeared to be an effort to wipe off much of the blood prior to our arrival, but I could see it went further down her body.

In the middle of Amy's abdomen were staples, which began just below her sternum and continued all the way down to a few inches below her navel. In her torso were chest tubes stuck into both sides of her ribcage. Her frail, petite body literally looked as if it were the victim of a shark attack or some other wild animal mauling. The reality of how she looked at that moment is almost impossible to exaggerate. In short, there was nothing any of them could have told me to prepare me for seeing her this way.

It seemed so ironic, so perverted and so unfair that someone as peaceful and easygoing as Amy had suffered errors that resulted in such violent trauma. The fear that surfaced in me was unlike anything I had ever experienced, and it took maximum effort for me to keep my composure. This version of medicine was an absolute butchery.

How fortunate we were that I had not seen Amy before I took time to pray. Sometimes a person can see something so shocking that rationale and clear thinking fly out the window. This was plainly one of those sights. Amy's horrifying appearance would have been distracting enough to prevent me from seeking prayer. Since she looked more injured than I could have ever imagined, the horror of seeing her that way might have been an obstacle too huge for me to overcome, seeking prayer. Not that this would have minimized my belief in God's ability to save her, but it may have prevented me from taking that opportunity to practice my faith in Him and mobilize others to pray for her. This was the terrible reality of what she went through, and it jarred me to the very core of my being.

The nurses who were present told us that they would be moving Amy to a room on the eighth floor in the ICU ward. Ushered by the same nurse who took us back there to see her, Helen and I reluctantly left the recovery area so that the nurses could finish up prepping Amy for transport.

Our return to the private waiting room revealed to everyone who was present that the situation was grim. There were so many questions to be answered, but no answers to be had - at least not at this time.

Amy's sister, Crystal, called Dalton, my father-in-law, on her wireless phone and he wanted to speak with me. Although not in the mood to speak to anyone, I took the call anyway, recognizing that I had more information about the condition of his daughter than any of the other family members. If there was bad news to be given - and indeed there was - then I should be the one to relay it.

I took the phone and Dalton, who was working and would not make it to the hospital on this day, asked me what was going on with Amy, except he didn't word it so diplomatically. There was no question that he was furious. It was apparent that he had gotten word from someone else about some of the events that had happened, or the condition of his daughter, or both. I answered his question by telling him that Amy was in bad shape. Our phone conversation was short and before we ended it, he asked me if I was *"in good with the Lord."* I didn't understand him right away because what I *thought* I heard was so out of character for him, so he repeated the question. When I replied affirmatively, he told me to concentrate on praying for his daughter, because his own concerns were on - well, I'll just say he used the words "doctors" and "shotgun" in the same sentence.

The conversation with Amy's dad added stress to the matter. He loved his daughter, and it wasn't a stretch to believe that he would arrive at the hospital ready for a fight. In any instance, I couldn't blame him for the ferocity of his anger over Amy by wanting to antagonize those who were responsible for putting her in this condition.

It seemed like a very long time before Amy was moved from recovery. It was between 6:25 and 6:45 p.m. when they finally moved her to a private room in the ICU, and those of us still in the family waiting room were escorted to the ICU waiting area on the hospital's eighth floor. The room that Amy occupied retained a cold temperature, had dim lighting, and was positioned directly in front of the nurse's station for priority monitoring. I suspect the hospital staff knew that Amy got a raw deal in terms of medical care. They could do nothing less than to prioritize her treatment from this moment on.

The ICU waiting room had fewer people in it than the surgery waiting area on the lower floor, and it was more comfortable than that area as well. The seating area was carpeted, and the windows were tinted. Vending machines were on the floor and other small conveniences. The ICU waiting room was more tailored for families who might find themselves staying longer than the other visitors elsewhere in the hospital.

By the time she was moved from recovery, Amy had undergone the equivalent of 3 major surgeries. We were assured that the doctors had done all they could. Her body's own healing ability came into play, but a person was not designed to sustain this kind of trauma in such a concentrated period of time. There was no sense of optimism from any of the physicians, hospital staff or anyone else for that matter. The only thing I had to hang onto was the hope that God would perform a miracle for us.

Life support machines and monitors were around the hospital bed that held Amy. She had tubes and wires all over her. A ventilator breathed for her and many other devices were present to aid in life support. A tube was down her throat and tubes went into her nostrils. A catheter had been placed to monitor urine output. Chest tubes were present on both sides of her torso, with two inserted on her right side; one on her left. There were lacerations on other parts of her body as well, but those wouldn't become visible to me until much later.

On her legs were inflatable hoses which filled with air to stimulate blood circulation to that lower part of her body; underneath those were fabric hoses that left her feet exposed. There was a catheter drip bag attached on the side of the bed and IV drips were there as well.

It would be a while before the remainder of those who had arrived earlier in the afternoon would begin to leave. Amy's condition interrupted the life cycle for everyone who managed to make it to the hospital. They would leave and go their separate ways to tend to matters they postponed to be present with us.

While everyone else was departing, a friend from work arrived at the hospital and found me in the ICU waiting room. How surprising it was for me to see Nash at the hospital to offer me his prayers and support. He was several years older than I, probably in his mid to late 50's. Nonetheless, at this particular time I had no better friend; he probably drove 30 miles to get to the hospital from where he lived. He came to the hospital to let me know that he was informed by our work supervisor of my situation and wanted to know if there was anything he could possibly do for me. I asked him to pray and to put Amy on the prayer list at his church. Nash, being the good Christian friend that he was, was obliged to fulfill my request and told me not to hesitate contacting him if I needed anything more. Over the days ahead he would routinely call to check up on me.

As the evening turned into night, only Helen and I remained at the hospital by the time my sister, Robyn, and her husband, Chris, arrived from the pastor's convention to check in on us. Chris called me on his wireless phone just minutes before to inform me that they were on their way to the hospital. I provided him directions on how to find us once he made it there. Without any problems, they made it to the hospital and found us in the ICU waiting room. They greeted us with hugs and told us they had already shared information about our situation with some of their pastorate friends. We learned that Amy was already on many church prayer lists.

We talked with Robyn and Chris for a few minutes about Amy, updating them on her condition. They were astounded at the idea that two separate mistakes had landed Amy in this predicament, fighting for her very life. After our brief talk they wanted to see Amy. I led them into the ICU room where she was being kept.

As if my words had done nothing to prepare them for what they were going to see, my sister and brother-in-law were stunned when they saw Amy for themselves. It was unbelievable to my sister that Amy could be so critical in such a short period of time. It had been only a few days earlier when she last saw Amy as her regular, normal self. For them to now see her in this way was a contrast almost too great for comprehension

Robyn and Chris asked us questions and Helen and I answered what we could. We didn't know the full extent of Amy's injuries or any specific details on how they happened or why, but we tried in desperation to put it all together with the pieces of information that we had.

As Robyn and Helen continued talking, Chris and I walked out of the ICU and back into the waiting room area. On the way back, we talked about the severity of Amy's injuries and though he knew I had other concerns, he steered the conversation towards the topic of legal representation.

Chris was the first to bring up the matter of legal consultation. He was aware of prior incidents that happened with regards to Amy's medical treatment by Dr. Keel. Before my discussion of this with him, I had not taken the opportunity to think about legal representation. My concern for Amy blinded me to thinking beyond her current state; although I was caught off balance that this was brought up as an option, I would later come to understand the wisdom of my brother-in-law's foresight and suggestion.

"You ought to think about contacting an attorney," Chris said to me. He talked about protecting my interests in this situation, explaining how Christians sometimes are often too willing to overlook matters where we are personally harmed. He commented that in doing so we can do ourselves a greater disservice, especially in circumstances so extraordinary. He also added that if it were he in my situation, he would take the initiative to get legal representation because Amy deserved better medical care than what she received. He assured me that this course of action had little to do with offending the doctors or the hospital, but it had everything to do with me protecting my wife. He said that an attorney could investigate the incidences leading up to Amy's injury and determine if these were honest mistakes or blatant negligence.

Because he is a pastor, I always took Chris's counsel at heightened value. At first, I didn't think much of his suggestion about hiring attorneys, but the sincerity and concern he projected eventually stirred my attention. He told me there was a member in his church whose daughter lived locally to us. She was an attorney and so was her husband. Chris offered to make a call on my behalf to get the ball rolling, reemphasizing that the decision was solely mine.

I thought for a moment. I really didn't need any additional concerns right now, no more than I needed to be worried about Amy's dad arriving at the hospital with his shotgun. I feared legalizing this predicament would make matters worse for Amy and distract the physicians and hospital's ability to provide her the best care, albeit at this point the care had been substandard for my wife.

My delay in responding to my brother-in-law may have made me appear quite indecisive, initially. But I wanted to make sure I was making the right call. People who filed malpractice complaints were without merit and frivolous complainers, *or so I had believed.* Popular beliefs about malpractice victims led me to deem they were all part of an elaborate scam to damage the medical industry for the benefit of lining their own pockets. Would I really become one of these people? *Talk about being naïve.*

What if those who complained of medical injury *really were* victims? What if these people actually have legitimate, legal complaints? In a moment, I realized that I was undergoing a tremendous paradigm shift in my own error-laden thinking about malpractice claims. My stronghold of personal pride began to topple from the foundation up, as it suddenly made sense to me that Amy absolutely did deserve better medical care than what she thus far received – that we both deserved better than what we received.

"Yes. Make the call," I told him.

I knew in my heart that I really didn't want it to come to this. I was not yet angry, for my concern for Amy still dominated my thinking. The anger would come later, but at this moment felt compelled to do everything I could to protect her. Maybe an attorney at my side would possibly help me to do that.

My affirmative answer to Chris about having an attorney notified was driven by another factor that also began to tear at me. Amy was on record as being an organ donor and it was my concern that the best efforts to treat her would fall short for the sake of harvesting organs. In my state, organ donor participants have this designation issued on their driver's license, so organ donation would be an indisputable matter in the event Amy died. It was my thought that an attorney would assist me to ensure that Amy wouldn't fall victim to a lack in effort of adequate treatment for the purpose of harvesting organs.

If Amy's organs began to shut down and system failure resulted (as Dr. Ferris seemed to think could happen) then organ harvesting might not have been possible, but I didn't recall this at the time. There was simply just too much at stake and I needed to do everything I could to protect her and look out for our interests.

Still, I was hopeful I did the right thing by allowing Chris to contact lawyers for me. I figured that if this were the right decision, then the wheels of justice would begin turning without too much additional effort on my part. Only the days ahead would tell if I was correct.

My sister and brother-in-law let me know that they would continue to pray for us and offered their assistance if we needed anything. It was late in the evening when everyone departed. My mother-in-law and I were the only ones who stayed at the hospital the entire night, taking shifts between Amy's room in the ICU and the waiting room. I was too exhausted and too agitated to sleep, yet I still needed to somehow refresh myself.

The first night of Amy's stay in the ICU was a very long one. Every half hour, nurses came into the room throughout the night to check her. There were several things the nurses and doctors had to do to Amy. Earlier, the nurses had informed us of certain things that they needed to continuously monitor. At this point any specific treatment outside of the routine required my signed authorization. The doctors would not perform certain treatment requirements unless I signed a treatment authorization document giving them permission to proceed. This unquestionably was an effort to cover the hospital and physicians from further liability and made me solely responsible for any new treatment courses they wanted to pursue — a position I wasn't pleased to be in. Because the mistakes that had been made were so immense, my confidence in the medical practitioners waned and I was afraid that I would sign an authorization that could unintentionally result in the termination of Amy's precious life. I had to make sure I thoroughly understood the treatment to be issued before signing authorization and I hesitated every time.

One of the authorization documents for which I had to sign was for placement of a swan catheter in Amy's iliac artery — in the pelvic area — recommended by one of the treating physicians. Amy was experiencing *hypotension*, a severe and extreme drop in blood pressure. Her dangerously low blood pressure and swollen abdomen were sure-tell signs that her condition was not improving; in fact, it was getting worse. It soon became obvious that Amy's body was not responding positively to the surgeries. With all of the IV lines, catheters, and plastic tubes positioned in her, I presume the only place left to place this swan catheter was in her left iliac artery. The IV drip that was put through the swan catheter contained medicine that was supposed to aid in stabilizing or reversing her critically low blood pressure. Although we would not discover it until later, the attempted placement of this catheter would become the source of yet *another* injury to Amy.

Helen and I hovered over Amy when the nurses were out of the room. We touched her, held her hand, and talked to her — anything to let her know we were there. Her feet were exposed from the hoses that covered her legs and for some reason I touched her feet. There was a distinguishable difference in the temperature between her right foot and her left foot. I asked Helen to feel Amy's toes but didn't tell her why. I wanted to see if she noticed the stark temperature difference as well. Helen touched them both and wondered audibly why Amy's right foot was warm and her left foot was ice cold. There was nothing external that we could see causing this.

We pointed out the temperature variance between Amy's feet to the nurse assigned to her room. The nurse came in and checked for herself the concern that caused me to go get her. The nurse seemed baffled and examined the equipment. She looked under Amy's gown and underneath the bed. She had no answer as to why Amy's left foot was frigid compared to the other. When asked if we should be concerned, the nurse replied that she would look into it again, but there was really no reason we should be alarmed.

As the night moved on, I couldn't help but to become increasingly concerned about my mother-in-law, Helen. She was experiencing a parent's worst nightmare, having to cope with the certainty that she could lose her daughter. Helen was a bundle of nerves and would expend the next 14 days at the hospital. Like me, her trust in the hospital and the doctors was virtually nonexistent and she determined that Amy would always have at least one family member present. It was our hope that if Amy could not make it through this ordeal, then at least she wouldn't be alone.

My concern for Helen factored into my overall anxiety and I prayed for her as well throughout the night at every opportunity. Although extremely exhausted, my concern for Amy, Helen and the whole situation made rest impossibly elusive.

CHAPTER 9

Day 2: March 8

The early morning of March 8th greeted us with more doctors. I was introduced to a doctor by the name of Edwards who was contacted by Dr. Keel to assist and coordinate Amy's care through the remainder of her stay at the hospital. I also met doctors Wales and Milton, both vascular surgeons who had already operated on Amy. Dr. Wales' specialty targeted areas above or north of the diaphragm while Dr. Milton's specialty targeted the areas below or south of the diaphragm. Dr. Lister was the anesthesiologist who worked on Amy in one of the surgeries and he arrived early in the morning to check on Amy's prognosis.

The fact that Amy did not respond well to the overnight treatment initiatives led the medical doctors to conclude that Amy needed another surgery. No one was more unhappy about this recommendation than I and this news was met with resistance. How many times did it take for them to get things right? For the first time since Amy's hospital confinement, I vocalized my anger because I knew that with each surgery came the increased chance for another life-threatening mistake. They had already butchered her. Why weren't they satisfied that she had enough?

Dr. Milton told me that Amy needed the "re-exploration" and said that her chances to improve would fail without it.

The doctors couldn't perform the surgery on Amy without my authorization. I had to sign Informed Consent paperwork authorizing them to perform certain treatment and there would be other times in addition to this one where I had to give authorization. I obviously wanted Amy to recover, but I simply didn't have full confidence that these doctors knew what they were doing. Would I allow the surgery and risk the possibility that they could further agitate Amy's already fragile condition, or would I deny the surgery and just hope for the best? Family members who had learned of the situation offered their input, some wanting me to authorize the surgery and others recommending against it. But the decision to authorize the operation was clearly in my court. I had a very important decision to make.

I could approach my decision on whether to allow the surgery from two positions: The first was that of emotion. I *hated* the very idea of Amy going back under the knife. It was my understanding that the surgical errors had caused Amy's multiple injuries and the gamble of her having to undergo another surgery had the potentiality of another life-threatening error. Two had already been made; this was the *only* reason she was in critical condition. The second position was that of logic. The doctor claimed Amy needed to go back under the knife to improve her chances. He, being medically trained and practiced, was the one educated to make the recommendation, whereas I was not. I wrestled with not knowing what to do and again fell back on prayer.

Soon, I realized I had no choice but to trust the doctor's recommendation because it would – at the very least – shift some of the responsibility back upon the medical team. The entire time through this journey, Amy and I trusted the doctors; and although at this point, I did not have highest confidence in them, I knew of no other way to get through this except to try to trust the doctors once again. I wasn't happy about it, but my choice was made. Amy would have another surgery and it would take place within minutes of my signing the Informed Consent form.

It could be argued that my decision to allow the surgery was a lack of faith, but I would disagree. Faith is never exclusive from action. Faith motivates action whereas lack of action is simply giving up. I remembered the faith without works Scripture reference. Miracles often result from praying as if everything depends on God while working as if everything depends on you. In the case of Amy's survival, I never lost sight of the fact that in addition to ongoing prayer, we had to try *everything* we could to give her the best chance.

Helen and I were asked to go to the waiting room while the medical staff prepped Amy for surgery. As we exited the room, the curtain was drawn to conceal the room. Helen and I returned to the waiting room as asked and waited for the nurses to notify us before Amy would go into the operating room. It was during this time that I received a phone call into the ICU waiting room.

On this floor, there was no desk manned with someone answering phones like the other waiting room. There were phones on both sides of this room – which was separated by a hallway – and there were two other families occupying the area. One of the strangers answered the ringing phone and called out my name. I walked over to take the phone from the woman who answered it, not knowing who would be calling me.

I took the phone and identified myself. Someone that I had never spoken to before identified herself as Megan and told me she was informed that I needed the legal services of an attorney. Although surprised, I replied to her affirmatively. We had a short conversation over the phone that lasted no more than a couple of minutes. Megan was on her way to the hospital, and it didn't take long for her to arrive in the ICU waiting room, finding me sitting with my mother-in-law.

Megan introduced herself and as we began to talk, we were interrupted by a nurse who found and informed me that Amy was about to be taken into surgery. I excused myself and departed from the ICU, following the nurse to where Amy was. When I saw Amy lying unconscious on the hospital bed, I took a moment to gaze at her, wondering if she were aware of anything going on. Placing my hand on her forehead, I bent over to kiss her cheek. Her body felt so cold, and her skin was colorless and pale.

The medical staff moved Amy through the hall and disappeared onto the elevator that would descend to the level where the surgeries are performed. When Amy was out of sight, I returned to the waiting room and discovered two other people whom I didn't recognize sitting down and talking with my mother-in-law. Megan was still there, and the newcomers were men dressed in suits and they held legal pads. They had come here to talk business.

It was a very awkward moment for me when the attorneys were there. There was no subtleness in their appearance, and they stood out from everyone else. One of the men was the husband of Megan and the other man was his associate, a partner of a professional law firm in the downtown area of our city. These were the people who were contacted through my brother-in-law, Chris.

Another round of introductions were made and after assuring me that everything we discussed would be kept in strictest confidence, they implored me to tell them exactly everything that was happening. Helen and I obliged, informing them of everything we knew had happened up to that point answering as many of their questions as we possibly could. Amy's older sister, Crystal, arrived just in time to assist in answering questions and was a valuable resource in collecting and providing additional information for the attorneys. Obviously, I was uncomfortable having the lawyers there, but they provided beneficial information about our situation and gave me some things to do that very same day.

The attorneys told me that their experience with malpractice cases taught them that medical records have a tendency to become altered or "doctored" before anyone outside of the medical realm can view them. I was instructed to obtain Amy's records from Dr. Keel's office as soon as humanly possible. They also provided Helen and I with disposable cameras and advised us to use up all the film taking plenty of pictures of Amy and her injuries. They made it clear that this would be an essential part of building a case and added a request for me to maintain some form of confidentiality from the doctors.

The confidentiality request was a rather obvious one. I didn't want it known that I had spoken with any attorneys because I didn't want medical personnel distracted from performing their best while Amy was still dependent on their skill. I didn't want to form a bigger wedge between myself and any of the treating doctors or the hospital. I didn't want to appear to be taking advantage of a negative situation for my own personal gain. The last thing I wanted was to appear to be an opportunist; and equally, I didn't want to be perceived as an antagonist or a troublemaker. So, I imagined that it was to my benefit to try to maintain some sense of secrecy about any legal recourse.

Before leaving us, the attorneys gave each of us a business card and told us not to hesitate to call them if anything else came up. They also indicated that they would be in touch with me very shortly to obtain the records that I collected from Dr. Keel's office and to get the cameras from me. After talking with them I felt as if I had made the right decision in allowing them to be contacted. I felt as if Amy and I now had an advocate to help us answer the many questions that would inevitably arise; but at the same time, I was very relieved that the attorneys left when they did.

Sometime after the attorneys left, I received a call from the operating room, between 60 and 90 minutes after they wheeled Amy away. The voice on the phone told me that Amy was out of surgery, that she was stable, and that Dr. Milton would be up to talk with me soon. I anticipated another hour or so before I would see the surgeon. I was surprised that Dr. Milton arrived not very long after the call. He found me in the waiting room and came over to where Helen and I were and sat down.

Dr. Milton told me that things went well during the surgery and that Amy was responding positively to the intervention. He explained that she had additional internal bleeding in her abdomen that wasn't caught during the initial surgery. He added that he was also able to repair a perforation to several areas on her colon and a torn iliac artery on the left side of her pelvis.

When we inquired how these injuries were missed during the earlier surgery, Dr. Milton told us that the initial injury was deeper than they had realized, holding his fingers about 6 inches apart. He said that during the earlier surgery he repaired the vena cava, or the blood vessel closer to the surface of her abdominal wall, but the one he had just repaired was deeper than the first and was suspect to ongoing internal bleeding overnight. He also explained how the colon lays over itself several times and when the injury occurred, it shot straight through several folds; thereby perforating the colon in several areas on the surface.

I would come to learn that the iliac artery injury on the left side of Amy's pelvis occurred the evening before when a doctor attempted to insert a swan catheter into it unsuccessfully. This attempt damaged the artery and became an additional source of internal hemorrhaging. This would explain the reason why Amy's left foot was icy cold even though her right foot was warm. The iliac artery tear prevented ample blood from flowing to her leg. Because of the damage of the left iliac artery, the catheter had to be placed in Amy's right iliac artery.

I was notified by a nurse when Amy was returned into the ICU room from the surgery. Knowing that the surgery had been completed successfully without any complications only increased my desire to see Amy, and I didn't waste any time getting back to her room when they told me she had made it back.

Present in the ICU room that Amy occupied were a couple of medical personnel checking Amy over and taking some readings. When I saw Amy, I noticed that she looked very different now than the last time I saw her. Amy's entire body had swollen unlike anything I had ever seen, as if water had literally been pumped into her. She was so swollen, in fact, that I couldn't help asking the nurse nearby why Amy looked this way. The nurse replied that it was common for the body to swell after multiple, invasive surgeries, adding that the number of surgeries Amy went through had triggered this response and that the swelling would subside after a couple of days.

After the nurses and I finished speaking, I drew the curtain closed and began to take pictures with the disposable cameras furnished by the attorneys. I hated the very idea of doing this because it was an action of *throwing down the gauntlet*. There was no turning back for me after I began taking the pictures. I realized that I better get hopping on retaining Amy's records from Dr. Keel's office as well.

As the day progressed, Amy's dad eventually made it to the hospital. He was still riled about the events that injured his daughter, but he was in a somewhat better mood when he arrived. Perhaps his delay in making it to the hospital was a cool-down period for him. It was around lunchtime when he arrived and he brought us some food, knowing that we probably had not eaten. It would be another day or two before he forced himself to go into Amy's room to see her. Like my own dad, my father-in-law epitomizes the strong role of man. But the idea of Amy being in a state where she was dependent on machines to keep her alive was the chink in his armor. He's only human.

Sometime that early afternoon, Dr. Wales came to the ICU waiting room to visit the family. He was one of the vascular surgeons who performed the emergency surgery on Amy after it was discovered that the transfusion was killing her. He found me sitting with Amy's parents in the waiting room and came over to sit where we were. He was a middle-aged man who had a very serious look on his face. He was aware of most everything that went on with Amy and made the effort to talk with us.

Dr. Wales greeted me and introduced himself to Amy's parents. He started the conversation by saying that it looked to him as if Amy was doing better, and asked if anyone informed us of anything regarding the transfusion. When we replied to him that we were not given any specific details, he shared with us those things he probably felt we should have known. He began by telling us that Amy had sustained injury when a central line IV was placed into her neck for the blood transfusion and described his role in repairing her subclavian artery on the right side of her neck. He mentioned that another doctor helped him perform the operation and explained to us that because the central line had not been placed properly, the transfusion blood Amy received filled her chest cavity rather than entering her blood stream. He said this made it necessary for an emergency thoracotomy, which is a procedure that involves opening one side of the chest to drain fluid and relieve the pressure of fluid build-up; in this case, the fluid was blood from the transfusion. He also mentioned that the chest tubes were placed for ongoing drainage of blood fluid.

When he finished explaining to us this portion of Amy's medical intervention, Dr. Wales asked us if we had any questions, he could answer for us. I don't remember which one, but one of my in-laws took this opportunity to ask him how the error was made that caused the central line to be placed incorrectly. He hesitated only a moment, then answered by telling us the doctor who inserted the central line into Amy's neck apparently missed the vein and instead hit the artery, puncturing into and through it. The incorrect placement caused filling of her neck and chest with blood, which caused a gradual decline in her blood pressure to a dangerously severe degree, nearly irreversible. At this, he stood up and left rather abruptly. His quick departure indicated that he might have said more than what he wanted to, or more than he was supposed to.

Later that day – sometime in the afternoon – my parents arrived from out of town and my sister and brother-in-law returned to the hospital.

My parents wasted no time in their effort to see Amy. They knew she was in a tough situation, but they were shocked to see her in such a terrible state. Amy's body had continued to expand and there was a lot of dried blood in her hair. With the maze of tubes, lines and wires running all over her, my mother cried when she saw Amy. Mom held Amy's hand and asked me how something like this could happen. I didn't know.

After moments, we left Amy and retreated to the ICU waiting room. I began talking with my dad and brother-in-law, Chris. I told them that the attorneys arrived at the hospital, and they wanted me to secure Amy's medical records from Dr. Keel's office. I confessed to them that I was uneasy about going to the doctor's office to ask for Amy's records and asked them to accompany me. The doctor's office was on the opposite side of the hospital complex. We were able to walk to that building using the ground and below ground corridors.

It was between 3:30 and 5:00 p.m. when we were able to secure Amy's records from Dr. Keel's office. When I arrived and made my request there was no delay in getting the records to me. In fact, it seemed as if the office anticipated my request and had a copy of Amy's records waiting for me, as if they were expecting me to come and pick them up. I was really surprised to get them so fast, and I was glad I was able to get them without incident. I was also thankful that we didn't encounter Dr. Keel. My dad was furious with Dr. Keel and because he was with me, I didn't want him to start a confrontation with the doctor.

When we returned to the hospital's eighth floor from Dr. Keel's office, I saw one of the attorneys that stopped by earlier to get information from me. The lawyer saw me walking his direction in the hallway and approached me. I introduced him to my dad and my brother-in-law and told him we were just coming back from obtaining Amy's records and immediately gave the copies to him. The attorney accepted the records, saying it was good that we had obtained these promptly and he mentioned that he came back with their law firm's professional camera to get more pictures of Amy.

We walked into the ICU room where Amy was, and Helen was taking photographs of her with this big, almost oversized flash camera. The attorney told me that the nursing unit supervisor would not allow him to take the pictures of Amy, so he had to recruit Helen to take the photographs. I didn't like the fact that this was taking place, but I realized that there would be a whole lot of things I wouldn't like about *any* of the legal stuff. My mother-in-law continued taking several pictures and based on how fast the nurses were scrambling around it was easy to see they also were nervous that all this was happening.

When the attorney was satisfied there were enough pictures, he collected the camera and told us that he will be in touch with us very soon. After he departed, I returned to the ICU waiting room and discovered a lot of people there: my parents, Amy's parents, my sister and her husband, Amy's sisters, members of our church and the pastor from our church. It was an amazing sight to see.

Our church became an extraordinary source of strength and support during this challenging point of our lives. They sustained us in a way that can never fully be told, except to say that it would have been vastly more difficult to live through this without them.

Everyone made their acquaintance with everyone else and to know that there were so many people who cared about Amy and our situation was really overwhelming. They visited for about an hour or so, and except for my in-laws and I, everyone soon left. Others returned in the days ahead to check up on us and provide ongoing support and prayer. Words cannot express how grateful Amy and I are for their encouragement.

The evening of March 8th brought a more positive outlook on Amy's recovery. It was a moment that – despite her appearance and continued reliance on life-support – possessed a tangible direction of hope on her ability to survive. Her lab readings were getting to the levels where the doctors wanted to see. And although I didn't know how Amy would be once she regained consciousness, I was optimistic since there were no more surgeries to be performed – at least as far as we knew. Amy was far from being out of the woods, but at least now there seemed to be a path.

Sometime during that evening on the 8th, I was sitting in the ICU waiting room involved in a discussion with Amy's parents, when Dr. Keel came to visit us. It was late in the evening, sometime between 8:30 and 9:30; we were surprised because we really didn't expect to see any more of her, especially that late time of day. Amy's dad had already told the hospital administrator and the ICU charge nurse that as far as he was concerned, he did not want Dr. Keel laying another hand on his daughter. He said that Dr. Keel was the catalyst of all Amy's injuries, and he wanted her to have nothing else to do with Amy. I am not certain if my father-in-law's request made it back to the doctor, but I suspect that it had.

A nurse led Dr. Keel into the ICU waiting room where we were. The doctor sat down across from us. I don't remember exactly how the conversation started, but Dr. Keel came to re-explain the initial procedure again (this time emphasizing the risks) and brought us up to speed on Amy's current condition. She offered us an apology – in the sense that she was offering her condolences – not in the sense that she was accepting responsibility for Amy's injuries. Showing us her palms and shaking her head, she said she was sorry that this happened to Amy, modifying her apology with the statement, "but sometimes these things happen, and Amy is just a very thin girl." When I heard this, I felt as if I could bite, literally *chew* nails, and I glared at the doctor.

Dr. Keel's comment was outright absurd, considering that Amy was unconscious and relying totally upon the doctor's surgical ability to perform the procedure correctly. In qualifying her apology, Dr. Keel was obviously trying to redirect the source of Amy's injuries, and I interpreted the modifying statement as if she were saying – whether intentionally or not – that *Amy* was the reason the surgery was botched. There are few things more demanding of a slap in the face than one's wife lying helplessly dependent upon life-support and the doctor responsible for putting her there essentially saying that Amy's thin size is the reason all of this happened. The morning of the surgery, Amy was virtually the same size she was since she first began seeing Dr. Keel. Amy was weighed at every visit with Dr. Keel and never once was it mentioned at any time that Amy would have to be a certain size to impact success of the surgery.

When she finished talking, Dr. Keel wanted to know if we had any concerns or comments and invited us to be open with her. I passed on the chance to say anything because I really wasn't in the mood for the discussion with the doctor to turn negative, although in some respects the doctor had already taken the discussion there. My mother-in-law said nothing.

My father-in-law, however, looked sternly at Dr. Keel the whole time she spoke. He was very patient before responding. It was evident that he wasn't happy with what she was saying. His first response to Dr. Keel was a comment about getting attorneys involved to find out the exact truth about how Amy was injured. He wasn't buying the "hands off" explanation she was trying to sell. My father-in-law can be rather intimidating when he wants to be and he used this skill when talking to the doctor, probably to let her know he had no appreciation of her account of the situation.

Dr. Keel answered him, saying that if he felt it necessary to call an attorney, then that was certainly an option that was available to us. He looked at her squarely and told her that his feelings about lawyers were the same as his feelings about doctors. He then asked her what she called 30 doctors and lawyers jumping out of a plane. Dr. Keel paused before replying she didn't know. He enlightened her with his simple, one-word answer: *"Skeet."*

This classic reply to the doctor was almost hilarious – not because the topic was light, by any means. It was because the situation demanded a strong way to convey our thought about what she had told us, and he gave her a perfect one without swearing or even raising his voice. Had the situation not been so serious, this moment would have demanded an audience. If only for this single moment, I was glad he was there to – in his unique style – put everything back into perspective for the doctor, who left as quickly as she arrived. After Dr. Keel scrambled away, my father-in-law reiterated to me and Helen that he did not want that woman laying another hand on Amy.

After Dalton left for the evening, it would again be Helen and I who stayed overnight at the hospital. The ICU waiting room contained the families of two other patients receiving medical attention on this floor, and we made acquaintance with one of the families present there.

CHAPTER 10

Day 3: March 9

The next day emerged. Amy was still in the ICU, but we greeted this day with cautious optimism. Amy had slowly begun to progress, and the overall swelling began to subside. Her vitals stabilized and her waning health leveled off. These were the first substantial positive signs that Amy was beginning to improve.

Every morning, Amy received a visit from Dr. Edwards, the physician consulted to coordinate Amy's recovery efforts. His specialty was internal medicine and he always had at least two people with him, who were perhaps medical interns. As he made his rounds, Dr. Edwards updated me every morning on Amy's prognosis and provided his plan of care orders to the attending medical staff for each day. He was always careful not to appear overzealous about Amy's progress and seemed to emphasize his concerns over any progress she made. He probably didn't want to give us any false sense of hope that Amy was out of danger. We respected his approach to her care and his dealings with the family.

Amy was still sedated and still required the ventilator. She was still intubated (tube in throat to maintain open airways). She still had the chest tubes inserted into the sides of her ribcage. She still had the urethral catheter inserted and the inflatable hoses were still on her legs. She still had IV drips with medicine flowing into her and she still lay there, unconscious.

Dr. Edwards ordered daily x-rays of Amy's chest, so the hospital's x-ray technician arrived in the room to take his daily pictures. I assisted the technician as he worked to get the best exposures possible. I helped the x-ray tech to make sure Amy was treated gently, because even though she was unconscious, I wanted everything to be just right for her. The television mounted on the ceiling was tuned in only to the channels that Amy watched. *Golden Girls* was a favorite of hers. She also loved watching *I Love Lucy* and I made sure the attending nurses knew what her favorite stations and shows were.

Dr. Finch, who was the medical partner of Dr. Keel and practiced out of the same office, came in to see me. Dr. Finch informed me that Dr. Keel had gone away on vacation and that she asked her to check up on Amy. Dr. Finch seemed to be a calm and modest individual and I felt as if she had more of a genuine concern for Amy's situation than Dr. Keel. At any of the times that I spoke with Dr. Finch while Amy was hospitalized, I wasn't aware that she had assisted Dr. Keel in the operating room to correct the initial injury. Nonetheless, I was glad know that Dr. Keel was gone; and honestly, I didn't care if she ever came back.

The third day in the hospital brought additional visitors who were close to us and unable to arrive the day prior, including Amy's brother, Brent, and some people that Amy knew from her work. Apparently, the word had gotten out that Amy suffered injury in the hospital, and those who knew her wanted to know that she was going to be okay. For those who saw her only days before, the reality of Amy's current condition was shocking.

Strangely, this day seem to move much slower than the prior day. When a loved-one is in the hospital, there's nothing to do but wait; the waiting makes the time pass by very slowly. I tried preoccupying myself with reading, but instead found myself doing a lot of thinking of things unrelated to the text in my book. I thought about how upset Amy would be when she realized the extent of her injuries. I thought on how much discomfort she would be in when she woke up. I wondered if she would recover fully to be the same woman I married in the summer, roughly 9½ months earlier. There were so many thoughts jolting through my mind that I was again agitated and restless.

I found myself often going back and forth from the ICU waiting room to the critical care room that Amy was in. I sat beside her and watched as if she was going to miraculously open her eyes and start communicating with me. Later that evening, Amy did open her eyes for just a moment. Seeing this really excited me, but I knew in my heart that this probably didn't indicate anything significant, at least from a medical perspective. I had to realize that she was far from out of the woods; and as I looked upon her longingly, I noticed that her hair hadn't been taken care of. Considering the amount of machinery stationed around the bed it probably just wasn't a priority to any of the hospital employees.

I talked often with my mother-in-law, who spent as much time by Amy's side as I. Helen was extraordinarily supportive and continued trying to figure out how Amy could be the recipient of such treacherous medicine. She couldn't comprehend how all this happened to her daughter while under the "care" of physicians. Her duty to nurture and protect her baby had surfaced and I knew that her presence was a rare but strong positive element of the whole experience. I had come to rely on Helen; we forged a friendship that any son-in-law would be fortunate to have with his wife's mother.

I maintained communication with various members from our church since they received news about Amy. Belinda was one of the caregiver counselors at our church and made frequent trips to the hospital. She was a close friend of Amy's mother and instinctively made her services available to the family. She was a great listener and perhaps the best counselor I've ever known. As she and I talked about some of my concerns, I realized that Amy would have to accept the fact that she would be disfigured on a very visible part of her body. This was something I simply didn't think about beforehand because I was solely concerned about her capacity to recover physically.

Helen and I determined that Belinda, should she agree, be the one to inform Amy about the staples down the middle of her abdomen and the trauma she sustained while under the anesthesia. Belinda agreed to help us in this and asked us to contact her when the moment arrived. Belinda's willingness to help was another small thing that made a big impact. How fortunate we were that she was generous enough to make herself available for us.

CHAPTER 11

Day 4: March 10

The third day of Amy's ICU confinement had passed. Overnight between the second and third day was the first night that I was able to get some halfway decent sleep. This being the fourth day of Amy's stay in the hospital arrived with no significantly good news, but no significantly terrible news either. Amy's condition was the same as it was the day before; no improvement...no deterioration. From this moment on, I was more content to believe that God's hand was on Amy. The doctors had already performed the invasive surgeries, now the wonder of the human body's ability to heal was in play and just as vital – provided there were no more errors made in Amy's treatment. I prayed continuously that no more medical errors would happen.

After refreshing myself from the night's sleep, I made my way over to the ICU. I entered Amy's room and saw a nurse looking at the information displayed on one of the monitors while she wrote something down on her clipboard. The nurse looked at me as she began updating me on Amy's condition, stating that Amy was stable, and her labs were positive. This was extremely good news. I asked the nurse if there was any indication of brain damage or other negative manifestations I should be concerned about. The nurse answered only by saying that Amy was under sedation to aid her recovery and added that the best method to determine if any cerebral damage occurred was to wait until Amy was removed from the sedation. I asked the nurse how long it would be before the sedation would be discontinued and she replied that since Amy was still dependent on the ventilator, she would remain sedated. Once Amy started breathing on her own it would be considered a major step in her recovery. Before departing the nurse told me that Dr. Edwards would be up soon when making his rounds to provide me any additional information I wanted to know.

A time later, Dr. Edwards arrived with his regular entourage and talked quietly with the nurse on staff. He came over into Amy's room and began looking her over and reading the charts in his possession. He began telling the nurse what his orders were for Amy's continued treatment and then started talking to me. There was nothing considerable in what he said about her clinical status that I can remember, other than the fact that he didn't give a negative prognosis by the way of anything new – just some things that they would have to watch out for.

After the doctor and other people departed the room, I picked up Amy's hand and held it. I looked at her and saw that the full-body swelling that was once prominently significant was now nearly nonexistent. I brushed her forehead with my free hand and by accident, I noticed how pretty and clear her skin had become. The volume of clear fluids she was receiving through the IV drips manifested a glowing, olive, nearly flawless tone in her skin.

Later in the day, there were moments when Amy opened her eyes. Family members who were present in Amy's room witnessed this and were excited at this development. I observed her opening her eyes again and compared to the first time, it was a longer duration and to me, it appeared as if she recognized me. She tried to get up out of the bed by lifting her head but was too weak. I asked her to relax and soon her eyes closed again.

Amy's father was made aware of the news of his daughter opening her eyes. He came to the hospital before but had resisted going in to see Amy in the ICU; perhaps the exciting news made him reconsider. Although I was not in the room when it happened, I was told that he went into the room and left just seconds after his entrance. His visit was very brief, not longer than a minute or so; obviously, he was not prepared to see Amy in such a damaged state of being.

On the third day of Amy's hospital confinement, Dr. Edwards informed me that they were going to attempt to gradually bring Amy off the sedation. He ordered the hoses removed from her legs and the ventilator tube to be pulled. Amy's progress, nothing short of astounding, had everyone hoping for the best and the doctors appeared to be somewhat amazed at her medical constitution. I don't think any of them realized she had a real shot at recovering at all, let alone this soon. There was no additional concern conveyed by the doctors for permanent brain damage as was first believed, but no person was willing to claim that Amy would recover 100% or that there would be no lasting affect from the trauma endured through the mistakes made during her surgeries.

The removal of the hoses from Amy's legs revealed a massive swelling around the left knee. Comparatively, the left knee was easily twice the size of the right knee, which appeared normal. I was not looking for things to complain about, but it was just too obvious that something was wrong with her left knee.

The x-ray technician came in that morning to take the pictures of Amy's chest, just as he had done the prior morning. I was in the room again as the technician worked to get the pictures. I seized this moment to ask him to take pictures of Amy's left knee and explained why it was necessary to photograph it. The technician acknowledged that the knee looked injured and accommodated my request. He took 3 pictures: one directly overhead, one in front with the knee bent, and a side picture of the knee. The side picture was a tricky one for him to get, so I helped by holding the photographic back-plate while he angled the x-ray camera to get the picture. I thanked him for taking the x-rays and asked him how long it would take before they would be ready to view. He responded by telling me that within 24 hours the x-rays will be developed and interpreted by a physician.

The nursing staff told me that Amy was being given doses of pain medication through her IV's. As they prepared for her to come off the sedation, they told me that she would have the ability to self-medicate. I was anxious to be able to interact with her. It seemed as if an eternity for this moment to arrive, and by mid-afternoon Amy would awaken and be conscious for the first time since she came into the hospital.

Amy's mother contacted Belinda to inform her of the physicians' intention of awakening Amy that afternoon. Belinda unselfishly interrupted her schedule and drove the 35 minutes necessary to get from the southeastern quadrant of the city to the northwestern part. She was coming to perform what we had asked of her earlier and she arrived on time to assist.

Amy finally opened her eyes and was conscious for the first time since entering the hospital 3½ days ago. I was in the waiting room when this happened and I was alerted when she awakened, even though Amy first asked for her dad. This was a major milestone as far as I was concerned and a promising event that made me hopeful that she was further away from death's door. Amy's eyes were tired-looking and somewhat glazed, but there was no doubt that she was coherent and aware of what was going on. The nurse explained to Amy the button near her hand and how she was supposed to press it to receive more medication for pain; Amy acknowledged that she understood by weakly nodding, ever so slightly.

Family members present took their turns coming in and out of the ICU room where Amy had spent most of her time when she wasn't being operated on. I resisted hovering over her until she asked to see me. She was able to talk somewhat in a soft, quiet voice, but the tube that had been down her throat and now removed had somewhat impaired her speech, so it was hard for me to understand every single word. She was in pain – this much I understood. Amy could not lift her head or any other part of her body other than her arms, which were also limited in movement due to the IV insertions.

Amy was moving her hand around on the bed; when I realized she was looking for my hand, I took hers and held it. She looked at me for what seemed like a very long time. I could tell that she knew something was wrong, but she didn't seem to know how to ask. I told her that she gave us all a big scare and that I was glad that she was finally awake. She looked at me and tried to nod, then I saw her move her free hand and place it underneath her gown on the middle of her abdomen. I could see the question in her eyes as she looked at me and asked what was it that she was feeling on her stomach. It was here that I tried to explain that her surgery was botched and because of that she required a series of extensive surgeries to save her life. I then told her that Belinda from our church was in the waiting room, waiting to see her. I asked for her permission to leave so that I could let Belinda know that she was up. Amy affirmed my request.

Within a couple of minutes, I returned to Amy's room with Belinda and Helen. Belinda greeted Amy and told her how long we had waited to see her open her eyes. Amy gave a weak smile as Belinda leveled herself to the height of the bed and began to provide Amy known details of the ordeal that had happened over the past 3½ days. Amy placed her hand back onto her stomach as she looked at Belinda, who started to explain to Amy the metal that she was feeling with her hand were staples from one of the surgeries. Belinda asked Amy if she understood the information she had just received, and Amy nodded.

After everyone had departed, Amy became increasingly upset about the pain that she was in, the fact that she had lost almost 4 days in the hospital, and the realization that the surgery for which she came to the hospital for had not only been unsuccessful, but it also nearly ended her life. Amy kept pressing the button to receive more pain medicine into her IV drip and because Amy was pressing the button too often, the nurse had to limit the amount of pain medicine she was allowed to receive. Amy was upset at this and discouraged that nothing turned out as she had hoped. She knew that her life had been interrupted until she could recover – however long that would take.

As the evening turned into night and the night progressed into the pre-dawn morning, Amy struggled with the post-operative pain prevalent all over her body. As the sedation began to wear off further, Amy became somewhat more and more aware of her surroundings. She though she kept seeing spiders on the ceiling tiles in her room. The attending nurse said it was a common occurrence for patients coming out of sedation to imagine that they are seeing things not actually there. For Amy, this hallucination would soon give way to the dreadful realization of her injuries accompanied by the terrible pain she was in. It was about this time she told me she wished she had never gone through with the procedure.

CHAPTER 12

Days 5 – 16: March 11 – 22

The morning of the 11th, Amy began complaining of severe pain in her left leg while still in the ICU. Remembering I had already requested that x-rays be made of the left knee based on the significant swelling I noticed after the leg coverings were removed, I waited for the x-ray technician to come by to take more x-rays of Amy's chest, per the prior orders of Dr. Edwards. When the tech arrived, I asked him about the results of the x-rays of Amy's knee, to which he replied the results were negative. I asked him if he were certain, and he responded that the physician who interpreted the film verified it. I wondered why they never volunteered telling me this information if the x-rays were indeed negative, so I asked the same question to the attending nurse about an hour or so later. The nurse told me the same thing, strangely in almost the exact same words the technician had told me. After this, I didn't bring it up again until I saw Dr. Edwards.

That evening of the 11th, Amy's sister, Crystal, arrived back at the hospital to wash Amy's hair with waterless shampoo she purchased from the department store, along with a few other items that she bought for Amy's comfort. The volume of dried blood that came out of Amy's hair during the washing was tremendous, turning several of the hospital's thick, white, absorbent, terry-cloth towels into a dark, burnt, brown color. The fact that blood had been left in Amy's hair so long caused it to mat and it took Crystal roughly 90 minutes of painstaking detangling and combing to get it back to a near manageable condition. There seemed to be no concern on the part of the medical staff to have Amy's hair cleaned sooner, so when they finally got around to asking Amy about having her hair cleaned that morning of the 11th, Amy replied that she'd prefer to have her sisters wash her hair. In her mind, if it wasn't important enough to them to take care of it prior to now, then she would save them the trouble.

At this time, Amy was only allowed to eat ice chips. There were medical reasons why she could not eat solid foods at this time.

Amy's medical condition slowly improved to the point where she could be moved out of the ICU. On the morning of March 13th, she was transferred to the surgical ward on the eighth floor of the hospital. By this time, Amy was detached from many of the medical devices she was reliant upon earlier, but she still had the chest tubes inserted in her sides. Amy obviously still had trouble with her pain and as she complained of the soft tissue discomfort from the incisions, her left leg began to give her more problems.

Her level of discomfort made it nearly impossible for her to maintain a positive attitude. She remained as pleasant and polite as humanly possible to the hospital staff, but she was frustrated that they couldn't do more to address her discomfort. She listened more to the doctors than she talked to them, but she couldn't distinguish one doctor from the next. To her, they were all one in the same. Dr. Keel of course wasn't around due to her being out of town on vacation; Amy already commented to me that she didn't care to see Dr. Keel again.

Amy was dependent upon family for most of her non-medically related needs. She had finally come to accept her situation, however reprehensible it was. Her parents brought her in a DVD player so that Amy could watch some of her favorite movies, like *Steel Magnolias* and *Father of the Bride*. It was every family member's intention to make Amy as comfortable as possible. While we could do little to control her pain, we could at least try to make her surroundings a little more home-like. Plenty of flowers and gift plants from members of our church and other friends lined the west-facing windows of the 12 x 12 room.

Since Amy was moved from the ICU, I was able to transfer my makeshift bed from the ICU waiting room to Amy's new room on the unit floor. In it, the room had a reclining chair that made for a rather uncomfortable but sufficient as a sleeping apparatus. As I slept in her room at nights, I was often awakened by her crying and sniffling. I would wake up and ask her if there was anything I could get her, but most times she already had the call light triggered for a nurse or orderly to respond. Sometimes they came promptly, but most times they didn't. Amy's pain medication was wearing off too quickly and she wanted more and stronger doses of medicine to ease her pain. The nurses could do nothing to give her more medicine because they were following a strict medication regimen.

By this time, I began working a full-time workday again, so getting sleep was not a luxury, but a necessity to be able to perform at work. It was difficult sleeping in the room uninterrupted. There were times when I just lay there listening to Amy cry in pain and it angered me that they couldn't do more to make her comfortable. Part of Amy's problem was that she had an intestinal obstruction causing severe, colicky pain; this in turn caused her to vomit repeatedly, have constipation, fever, and dehydration. I knew that in the morning, they would begin trying to get her to ambulate or to walk about and not be bedridden. But I found myself wondering how they were going to be able to get her to do so successfully. In my mind, it would be a monumental task.

Mid-day on the 14th, Amy was informed that they were ready to pull her chest tubes. During this procedure, Amy was asked to roll slightly to the left, and her gown was raised. She was prepped for pulling of the tubes as they removed the tape and bandages around both insertion sites on her right side. Amy braced herself as the physician in one motion pulled out the tube from the forward position. Amy gasped as the doctor moved his hand to the tube positioned in the back and pulled it. They quickly dressed and bandaged the wounds. Next, Amy was positioned onto her right side and she, holding onto my hand, squeezed it as the left chest tube was extracted. This wound was dressed and bandaged similarly as the other chest tube wounds on her right. The extraction of these tubes was a painful ordeal for her. Imagine an instrument with a ¾ to 1 inch diameter being stuck through your ribcage and into your inner chest, left for several days, then being pulled out on a moment's notice. What a tender area on a person's body to have this happen. It was not a pretty sight and seeing her in such pain made me weak.

In my absence, Amy's room was always accompanied by another family member there by her side to aid her efforts to get through this. The fact that there was always a family member around showed the hospital that we were not making light of Amy's care or her medical treatment. The doctors would never have to search for anyone to provide medical updates to. However, there was an incident that occurred with Dr. Milton on the 14th, when he asked that the family depart the room for reinsertion of the nasogastric (NG) tube that they removed on the 11th.

The NG-tube is a tube that is passed through the nasal passages and into the stomach. Amy was having emesis; that is, she could not keep anything down in her stomach and kept ejecting contents, even with only a liquid diet. Because this was so, Dr. Milton decided it best to reinsert the NG-tube. His first attempt at placing the tube was not successful, so he asked that family members leave the room so that our presence would not be a distraction for Amy. The people present were Amy's mother, Helen, my sister, Robyn, her husband, Chris, my parents, Michael and Brooke, and Amy's best friend, Karyn. Everyone, including myself, left the room as the doctor asked because we did not want to stifle the progress of Amy's medical treatment. We left the room and congregated in the unit waiting room not very far from Amy's room. There, we all waited until receiving notice from the doctor that they had accomplished their task and we could return to the room.

Dr. Milton emerged and found me standing alone in the waiting room, looking outside the eighth floor windows. He came over to me and began telling me how he was able to get the NG-tube in, but Amy had pulled it out. I asked him to repeat himself. He did, saying Amy pulled out the tube after he was able to get it placed and since she had pulled it out, he was going to interrupt her liquid diet to limit her emesis. I acknowledged what he had told me and asked him to share this information with the other family members, who were conversing with each other. At this time, I made my way back into the room and found Amy crying and in tears.

I kneeled to ask her what was wrong. She was visibly upset and very mad, saying the doctor held her down by her chest with his elbow and again by her neck while the other orderlies or nurses held her arms as the doctor tried to force the tube in. She said that after they released her, she pulled it out and threw it at the doctor because of the way they tried to shove the tube in; she didn't appreciate that. I asked her if she were certain she just didn't misinterpret what happened, and she told me to look at her chest. Her chest was red, as well as her neck. She asked me why I left her alone. Disappointed with myself that I had left her alone, I hugged her and apologized, agreeing that I should not have left.

Those who were outside the room began to filter in and realized that something was wrong. Someone told me that there were other visitors in the hospital in the waiting room asking to see me. Satisfied that Amy was calm enough for me to leave the room I found in the waiting area Frank and Steve, the attorneys I hired to take on our case. After greeting them, they asked how things were going and I updated them on Amy's medical progress. They asked if she was talking and able to communicate because they wanted to see her. I had them follow me.

We entered the room and I introduced everyone present to Steve and Frank and asked everyone to step outside the room while they took a moment to talk with Amy. After it was only just Amy, me, Steve, and Frank in the room, they began by introducing themselves to Amy. The summary of what they told her was that I hired them to investigate what happened with her surgery and to find why things didn't go as planned. They told her that they knew she was upset about a lot of things and said they were upset too. They told her that it was their job to make certain that she would be taken care of as she tried to make it through her ordeal. They assured Amy they would do everything in their power to see to it that those responsible for her injuries would pay. At this, they told us that they would be working on our case immediately and departed after excusing themselves. Though the visit didn't last very long, the timing couldn't have been better.

I felt betrayed by Dr. Milton because of the incident that happened with Amy when I was out of the room, and I wished I had another opportunity to see him so I could confront him. My first notion was to voice a formal complaint with the hospital's Administrator, but time helped me to calm down. The last thing I wanted was another adversary in the hospital, so while I could have raised a big stink about the incident, I chose to let it slide for the time being. But out of this, I further resolved to not allow any medical personnel treat her in any shape, form or fashion, without me or any other family member being present. Apparently, it wasn't enough that family was simply around. We had to make sure we were present *while* treatment was being conducted.

On the 15th and 16th, Amy worked with the physical therapist to try walking. She was not able to stand upright enough for this effort to be of much benefit. She was, in fact, totally dependent upon the therapists supporting her entire weight because she could not place any of it on her legs. Her left leg was very swollen and was so much trouble for her that we requested an icepack for her knee. No medical member wanted to address this and determined in my effort to try and understand what was going on with her knee, I commented aloud about her straining it once in a former job, but never having any additional issue with it before this time. This comment was apparently overheard by one of the medical workers, because it would resurface again in Amy's medical records and again in our lawsuit production responses.

Through the 19th, Amy continued to work on therapy and ambulating; there were two separate incidences where the practitioners working on her allowed her to fall. She was allowed to take a shower there in the room, but because she could not stand, she took the shower seated on a chair underneath the shower head. One of the staff nurses assisting with Amy's therapy seemed quite impatient and told Amy that having a baby was a lot more painful than what she was currently experiencing. I looked at the nurse and asked her if she ever had 4 major surgeries within a 24-hour period, and the nurse, sensing the point I wanted to make, instead said that she meant no disrespect, but she wanted Amy to concentrate on trying to get the most out of her therapy so that she could perform somewhat independently once discharged. I replied to the nurse that I was sure that no one wanted that more than Amy, herself. I reminded the nurse that Amy still had staples in her stomach and weakness in her legs and I told her I doubted any pregnancies resulted in such damage.

The nurses and therapists alike felt that Amy was not putting forth a strong and sincere effort to work on walking. They voiced concern that she was weary, not really motivated to participate in her physical therapy. Of course, all of this presumes that Amy's lack of enthusiasm was only mental and not physical. Amy knew that her body was not working well enough to get through the therapy, as time would prove that the damage was far more extensive than those medical personnel working with her were willing to acknowledge.

On March 22nd, Amy was promised an opportunity to be discharged. To get her prepared to go home, they had to remove the zipper-like, metal staples from the center of her abdomen. The medical worker used an instrument that resembled scissors, only the tip was different. This instrument wasn't designed to cut. Amy had as many as 60 staples down the center of her abdomen; she cried as each one was pried from its position. This was more terrible for me to watch than the extraction of the chest tubes, because it was a more painful experience for Amy where she had to endure the removal of 60 individual staples.

At this time, Dr. Keel arrived in the room, and I was surprised to see her because no one had seen her for several days. She had, I suspect, just returned from her vacation for which she departed on March 9th. Dr. Keel volunteered some information about Amy's medical situation and offered additional advice. I was too preoccupied to remember much of anything she said. But one question left me curious; Dr. Keel asked me if we attended church. I told her that as far as I was concerned, it was only the prayers of our church and many others that helped Amy live through this. Dr. Keel then made a comment about Amy's depressed mindset and offered to provide prescriptions to address this. I told her that Amy would be better once she got home to her usual surroundings and not wanting to linger at the hospital for any more time than what was necessary, I began to take the gift items that had accumulated from the eighth-floor room, out to the car.

Dr. Edwards authorized Amy's discharge pending an okay from Dr. Milton, who was the final doctor to okay her discharge. Final instructions at discharge included an effort for Amy to walk several times a day, gradually increasing activity and using the walker as needed; to keep Amy's incision wounds clean with soap and water daily, with a call to Dr. Milton should the incision wounds become tender or weepy; for Amy to use the spirometer daily, to increase her consumption of foods and to take one 7.5mg tablet of Lortab every three to four hours as needed for pain.

Finally, we were verbally instructed not to let Amy take any baths to help keep her wounds clean and to prevent against infection, tenderness, and weepiness. Dr. Keel opined in opposition to the nurse and told us that Amy could take baths as often as she needed. The nurse and Dr. Keel agreed to disagree on the matter. After this incident, I asked the nurse to see what she could do about getting Amy a walker for home use so that she could use it to assist her in ambulation. Then I departed the room to go pull the car around to pick up Amy from the hospital exit.

While in the elevator on my way down to the ground floor, I overheard two nurses I didn't recognize discussing the situation surrounding Amy's botched outpatient surgery and two-week hospitalization. Not realizing that I was her husband, they continued talking, one of them commenting to the other that the doctors thought Amy's pain and inability to walk were "mentally manifested" rather than actual lingering results of her many surgeries. The nurse who was talking then asked the other nurse if she thought the woman was really injured or just faking it for the inevitable lawsuit to follow. The second nurse scoffed and replied that if something similar happened to her, whether still in pain after the two-week hospitalization or not, she would sue just based on the fact that the first outpatient surgery wasn't performed correctly, resulting in the following surgeries and a two-week stay in the hospital. The elevator stopped on the second floor and the nurses exited, leaving me there to think about what was said. My first reaction to this conversation I overheard was how widespread the news surrounding Amy's situation had become within the hospital; my immediate second reaction was to ponder if those involved were withholding critical information due to an obvious suspicion that a lawsuit was brewing.

Helen was with us more than anyone else during Amy's occupation in the hospital and she was the one present with us at Amy's discharge. As I was pulling the car around, Helen learned that the discharging nurse was furious with Dr. Milton for wanting to deny Amy a walker for home use, for whatever reason. Perhaps he didn't think Amy was injured enough to need it, or maybe he thought the charge for it was coming directly out of his pocket. Whatever the reason, the nurse convinced Dr. Milton to sign for it. I did not find out about this incident until sometime later, after we left the hospital.

What an arrogant, unprofessional dip-wad Dr. Milton had shown himself to be.

CHAPTER 13

Rebuilding an Injured Life

After Amy's hospitalization, there were so many things medically wrong with her that we were forced to seek additional medical help. But with it being so soon after her hospitalization, we put off seeking medical help right away. We just weren't in any hurry to begin seeing doctors again.

Amy's daily pain management was difficult to get under control. Her sleeping patterns were sporadic. Her left leg became more of an issue. Her nutritional intake was not increasing. She still could not walk; her right eye was visibly injured, and the eyelid drooped. We allowed several days to pass to see if Amy could recover from with these issues on her own, but it wasn't long before we concluded that she would indeed need more medical attention. We tried putting off seeing more doctors, but Amy couldn't put off getting relief from the pain and I couldn't put off finding an end to watching her live through her own personal hell.

Amy's first specific request after being discharged from the hospital was to go to church on Sunday, March 25th. She had her own reasons for wanting to be there. Certainly, she was grateful to be alive, albeit with the pain. She knew about the many visitors from our church who had gone by the hospital to offer their support, even if they couldn't personally meet with or see Amy. She knew that these people had prayed for her and made her situation a priority in their prayer lives. She wanted to show these Christians that their love had sustained her. In church, Amy sat with me near the front. She couldn't sit up, so she lay on her side and listened to the singing and sermon. Pastor Johnson had come by to show us how glad he was to have Amy present in church. Amy knew it was paramount for her to be there that morning, to let everyone know that she wasn't giving up.

The first few days at home, Amy had the benefit of having friends or a family member sit with her while I was away at work. They saw first-hand how incapacitated Amy really was and upon my arrival, would update me on matters pertaining to her mood, comfort, and activity. When I was home, I noticed how reliant upon me Amy had become; I would have to cater her every need. She couldn't get from the sofa to the bathroom without help. She didn't have much of an appetite and ate only very small portions when she did eat. She kept watching the clock to take her pain medication every third hour. She would not let me get out of her sight without getting nervous. She was borderline depressed and at times would have moments of panic attacks.

When lying down, Amy would often lie on her back with a pillow behind her right shoulder blade. If she had to lie on her side, she would always favor the left, because the only wound on that side was that from a single chest tube entry. Her right side had more wounds, so she tried to avoid lying on that side altogether.

On the 28th, Amy felt she didn't need anyone to continue coming by to sit with her. Nothing had changed in her physical condition to warrant this, but Amy wanted to give it a try to make it on her own without anybody being there. She was disappointed that she couldn't interact with people while they were there watching and assisting her. Prior to my leaving for work that morning, I made sure that she had everything she needed at bedside so that she wouldn't have to get up unnecessarily. I called home several times a day to check up on her; her situation was always unchanged.

On March 30th, I arrived home around 8:00 in the evening. I unlocked and opened the door to our apartment and realized that the entire place was dark inside. No lights were on; no television; nothing. As I began to assess the situation, I called Amy's name into the dark and listened. I heard sobbing from the back part of the apartment, from the bedroom. I turned on a light in the living room, as to not walk into anything, and made my way to the back to switch on the bedroom light. I found Amy lying on her left side in the bed, in a fetal position, crying without reservation. Her face, red and wet with tears, was a picture of terrible suffering.

I embraced her and asked how long she had been this way and she told me pretty much all day. I could barely make out her words, but I asked her to tell me what to do. She didn't reply, so I told her that we would have to get her to the hospital. Amy cried harder when she heard this. I had to assure her that I was not taking her back to the Northwest Presbyterian Medical Center.

Amy asked me if I could help her take a shower first. I granted her request. Helping to give her a shower was a process that was slow and required a lot of effort. But the water seemed to give her some relief from the constant pain. When she indicated that she was finished, I helped her out of the shower and helped her to get dressed.

I don't remember why it took so long, but we arrived at the emergency room at University Hospital just before 11:00 p.m. We checked Amy in and then sat in the waiting room, as instructed. We waited, and waited, and waited. Amy arrived at the hospital with her walker and because of this I assumed that she would promptly be seen by a physician. However, the hospital appeared to be understaffed that night, so we were not given priority. As we waited Amy grew more and more weary. Every single chair in the waiting area had wooden arms, so there was no way for Amy to recline. Sitting up caused her pain and this was certainly the longest she had to sit up since the botched surgery. After more than two hours of waiting, Amy begged me to take her home because it was too painful for her to continue sitting. At around 1:49 in the morning, we left the hospital without checking out or Amy ever being seen or treated. I was angry at the hospital and angry about the situation. What a disappointing waste of time. What a total aggravation.

On April 1st, Amy's brother, Brent, was celebrating his 31st birthday with a lunch party for family members. Amy and I arrived at the party around 2:00 in the afternoon with anticipation of enjoying the event but ended up having to leave early because of pain in Amy's leg. She was in so much pain that upon our leaving, we drove directly from the party to the Lakeside North Hospital emergency room. This emergency room was quite further away than other hospitals near us, but due to our poor experiences at those facilities, it was worth the extra time required to get to Lakeside North Hospital.

After our arrival and check-in at the Lakeside North Hospital, Amy was seen by a physician after about a 45-minute wait. Dr. Drew Elliott was the treating physician. He asked Amy a series of questions. No doubt there were plenty of questions, because the stares that Amy received from people in the ER waiting rooms at both University and Lakeside North made it obvious they could tell something was wrong. Amy was very skinny, used a walker to ambulate and walked at a snail's pace as I held onto her should she lose her balance. She could not stand upright fully and had a frozen right pupil with a drooping eyelid and pale skin. I was concerned that Amy's appearance would lead people to think that I was an abusive spouse. Amy's appearance raised questions that required answers and I wanted to make sure the doctor had all the information he needed to isolate the issue(s) with her leg and properly treat them. Amy did not trust the ER doctor. It was not personal, for she didn't know this doctor from any other doctor she hadn't seen before; still, she failed to answer many of the questions he asked, so I answered the doctor when Amy did not.

We learned from this Lakeside North Hospital emergency room visit that Amy's patella had sustained a recent hairline fracture. With only two x-ray pictures, they were able to determine that Amy's knee had been injured. The fracture explained the mysterious swelling and the pain associated with the knee. Amy was discharged with an immobilizer. Amy was concerned that she was running low on her supply of Lortabs and asked the doctor to write her a prescription, but the doctor refused. He told Amy that she would have to get a refill order from her primary physician or the other doctors from whom she was supposed to follow-up with. It was apparent that the ER doctor was taking a defensive approach to Amy's treatment.

In learning about the fracture, I had two initial reactions: vindication and anger. I felt vindicated in the sense that there was finally a medical confirmation and reason for the pain, tenderness and swelling of this area on her leg. My anger in learning about the fracture prompted an email to my attorneys when we returned home from the emergency room. I found it appalling that the Northwest Presbyterian Medical Center staff employees tried to hide the knee injury from me, as if I wouldn't be smart enough to figure it out. It was here that I determined that we could no longer afford to deny Amy additional medical care. For all we knew, she could have been dealing with other issues that the doctors treating her during hospitalization didn't address. The following day, I contacted the office of our general doctor to schedule an appointment for Amy.

It was Monday, April 2nd, when Amy had her follow-up appointments with both Dr. Wales and Dr. Milton. During the visit with Dr. Wales, the physician expressed to us how very fortunate we were that Amy was still around. He explained how severely low her blood pressure was when he arrived to provide assistance and added that he had never encountered a situation where a person's blood pressure was so dangerously low for so dangerously long. Dr. Wales also commented how the medical profession resists using the term "miracle", but this was the only word he could use to describe Amy's unbelievable recovery. He asked if there were any lingering issues impacting Amy's ability to function independently and if I noticed her having any memory loss. I told him that I didn't know for sure about anything suspect to her memory but proceeded to tell him about Amy complaining of constant soft tissue pain on both sides of her upper body, her abdomen, pelvis, and left leg. Dr. Wales replied that it would be several months before Amy's soft tissue pain would subside and the best thing to do was to stay on top of the pain by regularly taking her pain medicine. I also brought attention to Amy's drooping right eye and how the iris was frozen. Dr. Wales looked at Amy and asked if she remembered him. Amy answered, saying she did not recognize him; she then asked Dr. Wales if she could have a prescription for more Lortabs since she was running low. Dr. Wales hesitated, then commented that the Lortabs could be habit-forming and encouraged her to take them responsibly. Amy then asked if she could begin taking baths. Dr. Wales told her that at this point he felt she could begin taking baths but told her to get a second answer on that from Dr. Milton during her visit with him, whose office was in the same area as Dr. Wales'.

Amy saw Dr. Milton directly after her visit with Dr. Wales. Dr. Milton greeted us and immediately ordered x-rays of Amy's chest and abdomen, which were taken there in the examination room in his office. Dr. Wales looked over the x-rays while we waited and came back in to examine Amy's surgical wounds. He commented that they were healing well. Amy, not wanting to waste any time, asked the doctor if this meant she could take baths. Dr. Milton responded that she was healing well enough to begin bathing again. He wrote out a prescription for Tylenol 3 with Codeine and encouraged her to try taking the new prescription rather than the Lortabs. Amy told him she needed the Lortabs for her pain and promised to take them responsibly, adding she would have the prescription for the Tylenol 3 filled.

After the follow-up appointments with doctors Milton and Wales, we had the new prescriptions filled. But Amy's ordeal was far from over. She continued to complain of the stinging and tenderness of her incision wounds, the throbbing soreness of her limbs, the piercing aching of her body, and the torrent of pain in her leg. She appeared to build some resistance to the medication she was relying on to help ease her pain. In fact, several times throughout the night of April 3rd, Amy was awakened from her sleep by her pain. Her interrupted sleep was accompanied by weeping and this happened at all hours of the night: 1:22 a.m.; 1:50 a.m.; 2:42 a.m.; 3:11 a.m.; 4:05 a.m.; 4:32 a.m.; 5:15 a.m.; etc. This pattern continued over the course of approximately 3 weeks. It wasn't until the night of April 29th that I remembered her sleeping the entire night without interruption of pain.

On April 4th, I arrived home from work at around 7:50 p.m. Upon my arrival, I found Amy again hidden away in the bedroom, lying in a fetal position on her left side, sobbing. When I entered the room she immediately began telling me that she had been this way since early afternoon and she was crying so hard I had difficulty understanding everything she was saying. She reached the limit on her daily dosage of medication. She repeatedly kept asking me why this was happening to her and asked me why she was not allowed to die. I hugged her and told her that it wasn't her time. She said that the pain was too intense and asked if she could have her leg amputated. Upon hearing this, I positioned her head between my hands and with her forehead to mine I promised her that those responsible for her predicament would pay for their crime. Amy then asked me what could be done between now and then to help her get through this; I replied that we'd seek additional medical help and pray in the meantime for her comfort and strength.

In this heart-to-heart moment, Amy told me that she took five baths throughout the course of the day. My concern about the water causing her incision wounds to soften immediately surfaced and I asked her why it was necessary for her to take so many baths in such a short period of time. I wasn't angry, but highly concerned, because bath water was detrimental to her wounds and the primary reason why the physicians discouraged her taking baths so soon after her surgeries. Even though the physicians cleared her to take baths at this point, I knew they never intended for her water exposure to be so extensive; and while I was not ready to get an acceptable answer for this supposedly irresponsible activity, Amy provided one. She said the warm water helped to soothe the constant stinging of the wounds and reduced the aching. The water gave her relief where the medication failed to do so. Still, the concern that she was tempting infection and weepiness of the surgical wounds was of high concern; I pleaded with her to limit her baths to only once a day. She cried more when I coached her on this but agreed that she would have to reduce her number of baths and tolerate the pain rather than risking a situation where she'd have to return to the hospital.

The days and nights continued similarly up to April 23rd. On this day, Amy requested a follow-up visit with Dr. Edwards, the physician specializing in internal medicine who treated her during hospitalization from March 8th through 22nd. We initiated this visit because of Amy's continuing soft-tissue pain along the incision wounds on her upper body and abdomen. At the appointment, Dr. Edwards examined the wounds to make sure there was no infection or issues with the healing. He determined that the wounds were healing properly and only added that her pain was simply the result of her surgeries and added, like Dr. Wales, that it would take a great deal of time for them to fully heal to the point that they wouldn't bother her as much. He tested Amy's breathing during this visit and ordered no other prescriptions for the pain.

Since her hospitalization, Amy avoided wearing bras because of the pain on her upper body. She was petite enough to successfully pull this off; it would be several more months before her pain subsided enough to where she could start wearing them again. She was still so frail and weak that she could only eat small servings of soft, non-heavy foods. And the predicament of her physical limitations started to weigh on her emotional health. Things that never bothered her before caused her to panic and have anxiety fits, such as if we ran out of orange juice or if she had to miss out on social events because of her injuries. She was still dependent upon the walker and had incidences where she fell trying to (without assistance) get from the sofa or bed to the bathroom or living room. On one occasion, I scolded her for not calling me to help, but she replied that she only wanted to be able to perform this seemingly simple task without any help.

While Amy had no specific gynecological issues before she started seeing Dr. Keel, she's certainly had them since. Her menstrual cycle was unpredictable and caused her additional related problems. Amy would need to have this aspect of her health addressed. How fortunate we were fortunate to have found a local OB/GYN physician who knew exactly how to treat his patients. We were introduced to Dr. Reysa through our attorneys who recommended that we allow him to become Amy's replacement gynecologist, based on quality references they received from nurses and other local contacts.

Amy's injured leg did not improve any, and in fact, was getting smaller in circumference around the thigh. After her emergency room visit at Lakeside North Hospital on April 1st, she was discharged with an immobilizer with instructions to wear it to prevent bending of the knee. But her leg pain wasn't concentrated just around the knee. It was all over her leg, and any amount of pressure on it was unbearable for her. This prevented her from wearing the immobilizer, though she made a good effort to leave it on. Something was going on with her leg other than just the fractured patella. Even though she was still just over 80 pounds, she would not put any weight on the leg and pretty much dragged it while trying to ambulate. And the pain associated with the leg caused two more trips to the Lakeside North Hospital emergency room: one visit on November 14th and another visit on May 18th – more than 24 months *after* her medical injury!

On April 27th, Amy had her first visit with Dr. Sanders, a D.O. family physician who had a general practice not far from where we lived at the time. Amy's real post-hospitalization recovery efforts began with this visit to Dr. Sanders, who provided a complete assessment of the many things that were wrong. The appointment ran from 11:00 a.m. to almost 1:00 p.m. Dr. Sanders was stunned when she first saw Amy, more revolted when she examined Amy and even more surprised when we told her the details surrounding Amy's condition. During the examination, Dr. Sanders was very concerned about the iris of Amy's right eye being frozen and the pupil not responding to light. Further concerns regarded the limited strength in Amy's extremities and no strength at all in the left leg. Dr. Sanders marveled at the fact that the hospital would discharge Amy in such horrible shape. We told the doctor every single concern of ours about Amy's health and the doctor took notes, paying careful attention to every concern. As the doctor performed her examination of Amy, she dictated her findings as the office nurse typed everything into the computer.

At the closing of Amy's visit with Dr. Sanders, the doctor said she was ordering all of Amy's medical records from the Northwest Presbyterian Medical Center and she provided us a list of referrals for Amy to see for further assessment: Dr. Hanson, a neurologist, was consulted to address neurological response concerns. Dr. Olsen, an orthopedist, was consulted specifically for the left leg injury. Dr. Vickers, a psychologist, was requested to assist Amy's psychological health, as Amy's sluggish state of mind caused her to cry during the examination. Dr. Porter, an OB/GYN Dr. Sanders referred us to for a routine gynecological examination and assessment. The appointments with these specialists were set for us by Dr. Sanders' office and these appointment dates and times were confirmed by phone calls to our residence from the respective physician's offices.

The first visit with Dr. Hanson was on May 23rd, at 11:30 a.m. This new patient examination and general physical evaluation resulted in physical injury discoveries. Dr. Hanson was thorough in his neurological examination. He asked Amy to press her foot against his hand and as she did, he felt almost no resistance. He repeated and then asked her to pull her foot against his hand, and again he felt no resistance. He then asked her to lift her leg off of the table, but Amy could not do as he asked. I watched as he took a metal instrument resembling a tuning fork. He placed the instrument on various areas of Amy's leg and asked if she could feel the cold instrument against her skin. Amy shook her head. Dr. Hanson then hit the instrument on a nearby table to make it vibrate. He placed it on areas of Amy's leg and asked her if she could feel it. Again, Amy responded negatively. He then took an instrument resembling a spiked wheel and rolled it over areas of Amy's leg and told her to tell him when she could feel the instrument. She felt the instrument on her foot and slightly above the ankles, but she could not detect the instrument on her calf or above on the side of her thigh. This was when, to my horror, I began to realize the depth of her injuries. This appointment with Dr. Hanson revealed that Amy had sustained nerve damage affecting vast areas of the left leg; capillary trauma on the right side of her head, suspect in causing the drooping of the right eyelid and the unresponsiveness of her right eye; functional, but limited strength in her extremities, and very limited strength, feeling, and function in the left leg.

At the end of Amy's initial appointment with Dr. Hanson, he gave orders for several MRIs of Amy's head, left leg, pelvis and lower back; he also requested a CT scan of Amy's pelvis and wanted follow-up visits, including one for an electromyogram EMG. According to WebMD, an EMG measures the electrical impulses of muscles at rest and during contraction. Nerve conduction studies, which measure nerve conduction velocity, determine how well individual nerves can transmit electrical signals. Nerves control the muscles in the body using electrical impulses, and these impulses make the muscles react in specific ways. Nerve and muscle disorders cause the muscles to react in abnormal ways. Amy's EMG took place at the Northwest Presbyterian Medical Center on May 30th. For her, this test was a painful series of electrical pulses on her left pelvic area and leg. From the EMG findings, Dr. Hanson concluded that there was indeed nerve damage and provided a referral to Dr. Talbot, a neurosurgeon. Dr. Talbot was consulted to assist in determining where the nerve damage was within Amy's pelvis and how to aid its repair.

The first-round follow-up visit with Dr. Sanders occurred on May 23rd, late in the afternoon. Dr. Sanders discussed with us the findings of Dr. Hanson and the next step in Amy's treatment process. The doctor recommended Amy begin taking Ensure to address her nutritional needs and weight issues; a prescription for pain was also provided. Another follow-up visit with Dr. Sanders occurred on June 1st, to review Amy's MRIs. At this visit another overall physical evaluation was given and additional pain medication was prescribed.

The neurological appointment with Dr. Talbot occurred on June 6th. Dr. Talbot is said to be the best at what he does in this part of the country and he offices out of a brand-new building in a northern part of our metropolitan area, a few miles further north than where we lived at the time. The appointment with Dr. Talbot was for assessing the nerve injury and for treatment consultation. The surgeon explained that he believed Amy had nerve damage in the left side of her pelvis; more specifically, the femoral nerve. The MRIs (ordered by Dr. Hanson) that he received were not detailed enough for him to interpret exactly where the injury was located, so he had Amy go to get another set of MRIs made at another diagnostic and imaging facility. Dr. Talbot informed us that, depending on how the new series of MRIs turned out, exploratory and possibly corrective surgery might be necessary.

Dr. Olsen, an orthopedic doctor and specialist in sports medicine, first saw Amy on June 11th, for assessment and recommendation for treatment. Dr. Olsen ordered x-rays and found evidence of a fractured patella nearly 30 days after the staff at Presbyterian Medical Center denied any findings on similar x-rays taken of Amy's left leg. Dr. Olsen discovered that the nerve damage was causing the onset of osteopenia in Amy's leg and said he could not address this until the nerve problem was resolved. Dr. Olsen detailed in his records why Amy was having such extensive pain in her leg. The nerve damage was contributing to degenerating bone mass. The quadriceps in her leg had started to atrophy or lose muscle mass. Dr. Olsen also detailed in his records how, because of the issues with her leg, her unbalanced walking had lead to issues concerning gait and lower back pain. Dr. Olsen provided us a referral to Dr. Anderson, a pain management specialist who practiced out of the local Spine Hospital, he promised to work out a physical therapy regimen for Amy in the meantime.

The OB/GYN appointment with Dr. Porter, for which we got a referral from Dr. Sanders, took place on July 10th. Amy went in and had the examination with the doctor while I waited in the lobby. At the conclusion of the examination, she came out apparently upset at Dr. Porter and mad at me for not accompanying her to the examination. Amy complained that the doctor told her that her injuries were known risks of a laparoscopic procedure. What we didn't understand was how he could make such a comment when we were still trying to discover the depth and scope of Amy's injuries from the botched procedure. I personally thought it was premature for him to make the comment and felt it was a callous, arrogant and ignorant response. How tough it was for me to know that any doctor could practice a specialty in medicine with such a lack of compassion. Today, hundreds of unsuspecting women and their husbands trust their wife's health to his care. Certainly, the doctor should have kept his opinion silent since he did not know the emerging discoveries of Amy's injuries, but the fact that he didn't suggests that he already made up his mind that regardless of the discovery he would be against us. Dr. Porter presented to be a challenge to our legal case, as I will discuss further in the *Expert Witnesses, Standards of Care & the Medical Code of Silence* segment of this book. Amy voluntarily discontinued seeing Dr. Porter.

On July 11th, Amy had her initial pain management appointment with Dr. Anderson. Like the other doctors to whom Amy had been referred, Dr. Anderson already had the opportunity to review her MRIs and other furnished medical records. At the appointment Dr. Anderson explained to us why the pain in Amy's leg was not being managed too well by the medications, saying that there was damage to the actual nerve tissue, which is an injury that does not respond very well to medication. He consulted with us over some pain management options and said he would contact us after further review of Amy's other records, which he would obtain from Dr. Hanson and Dr. Talbot.

On August 16th, Amy had a follow-up visit with Dr. Anderson. He recommended an electronic implant connected directly to Amy's spine to interrupt pain messages in her leg. Dr. Anderson provided a video and some literature describing the procedure and the documented risks, which included possible spinal cord injury, paralysis, headaches, infection, and should the implant device malfunction, it could cause pain rather than prevent it. Armed with this knowledge, Amy decided against having the implant and resolved herself to deal with the pain, just as she had been doing for the prior several months.

The counseling sessions that Dr. Sanders ordered for Amy with Dr. Vickers didn't begin until sometime the following year after Amy's medial error hospitalization event. With the multiple doctor visits that Amy was having throughout prior year, the 30-minute counseling sessions with Dr. Vickers simply wasn't possible, even though during this time I had secured an overnight position at a warehouse so that my days could be "free" to take and accompany Amy to her hospital visits.

In September, approximately six months later after Amy's botched surgery, she had an appointment with Dr. Brock, a disability examination doctor for the Social Security Administration to secure Disability benefits. Dr. Brock assessed Amy and his findings were consistent with that of Dr. Hanson, Dr. Talbot, Dr. Sanders, and Dr. Olsen. Regardless, Amy was denied the Disability benefits, which really devastated her. For those of you who clamored for government healthcare, denial is exactly what you can expect.

The news from the Social Security Administration denying Amy's claim for Disability benefits was a catalyst that triggered in her a crying tantrum, as if she had built up all this frustration over the months and was looking for a release. She was so worn by the process of seeing doctors, dealing with pain day-in and day-out, and the sleepless nights, that she started to feel as if all our efforts were in vain.

Our decreased household income did nothing to help matters any, and the occasional updates from our attorneys on the slow progress of building our case caused Amy more anxiety because it was apparent that many of the practitioners involved in her treatment during her hospitalization weren't making the discovery process easy. The defense was going to fight us at every point in this legal contest. What I thought would be a no-brainer concession by the defense based on Amy's obvious injuries was turning out to be a war of the wills. The only hope we held onto during this extremely low point in our lives was the knowledge that God knew what we had survived, what we were struggling through and the fact that we did not ask for this fight. We would have gladly settled to spare the upcoming battle and the stress it brought, but no party from the defense was willing to come forward to spare us the legal challenge.

Dr. Olsen, the orthopedic doctor, set up rehabilitation sessions and physical therapy for Amy at the McConnell Outpatient Rehabilitation Center. In the latter months during the year of Amy's botched surgery, she had 45-minute therapy sessions throughout the months of July, November, and December, and kept every one of them, treating them as serious steps in her recovery process. My mother-in-law assisted us by driving Amy to the therapy appointments on the days that I couldn't.

During the remaining months of that same year, Amy worked hard to regain her former life prior to her hospitalization. She had small successes, characterized by achieving and performing little tasks that she was unable to perform since before the botched surgery. For example, in early September of the year of the botched surgery, she was able to bend over enough to put on her own socks; although she was still dependent upon her walker to move about, she learned how to use it without falling. That same year, Amy and I attended the state fair in autumn. She took plenty of sit-down breaks and I had to give her a piggy-back ride from the parked car to the fairgrounds and back. This was the first extra-curricular event that we were able to attend since her medical injury.

On September 25th, Amy began wearing bras again. She admitted that it was uncomfortable for her due to the soreness, tightness, and tenderness of the soft tissue incision wounds on her upper body. But she said she needed to get used to it again. Hearing this encouraged me because it was a sign that her mental and emotional prospects were starting to look up. Her decision to begin wearing the upper body undergarment was a small personal victory in her long road to recovery.

Sometime between September and November in the year of Amy's botched surgery, she stopped relying on her walker. On December 19th, Amy and I went to the *North Mall* to look around, purchase a few gifts, and try to allow ourselves to get caught up in the Christmas spirit. We were fortunate to find a parking spot close to the southwest entrance even though the place was packed with shoppers and such. Walking through the mall, I realized how Amy's walking became more labored, slower and how her facial expression of excitement faded to that of concern. She was hurting and our stops to rest on the benches positioned throughout the mall became more and more frequent, with the first being only ten minutes after our entry into the mall.

The counseling sessions with psychologist, Dr. Vickers, were beneficial for Amy and provided an outlet for her to finally express her feelings about her situation in a manner that she wasn't perhaps able to before. Amy wept in her first meeting with the doctor; Dr. Vickers assessed that amazingly, Amy had a healthy spirit in spite of all the tragic events and degraded quality of life she had to endure. I do not know how the doctor came to this conclusion, but it was positive news for us and any good news we could latch onto was a steppingstone to a better future.

The horrors of Amy's medical injuries are real, and the evidence suggests a clear case of malpractice. While a few, self-absorbent physicians downplayed the true extent of her injuries, other physicians discovered that her injuries were far greater than normal laparoscopic surgery complications. This is an indication of gross negligence by the physician performing the surgery. The list of prescriptions alone adds measurable consideration to our injury claim: Hydrocodone 7.5mg; Skelaxin, 400mg tablets; Neurontin 300mg capsules; Acetaminophen #3 w/Codeine; Ultram 50mg tablets; Diflucan 150mg tablets. Additional injuries to Amy after the initial injury may have been avoidable and may indicate further negligence by other parties. We won't know the final results of the suit until trial occurs.

One of the most telling arguments for our complaint comes from the operative report dictated by vascular surgeon, Dr. Wales:

The patient is a 23-year-old female, who underwent laparoscopy earlier today with intraoperative injury of the inferior vena cava, repaired by Dr. Milton. A right central line was placed for fluid resuscitation. I urgently responded to the recovery room when a request for any cardiovascular surgeon was announced over the PA system. The patient was in extremis with marked hypotension and poor response to volume infusion. A right chest tube was placed by Dr. Hallund, and this returned a large amount of blood. Chest x-ray revealed a large hemothorax and the previous chest x-ray revealed an abnormal central line position and course through the mediastinum. The difficulties with hypotension and marked neck swelling began after the central line was removed. The patient was in extremis at this time, and I took her immediately to the operating room with ongoing resuscitation for an exploratory thoracotomy.

Is there any doubt of the severity of the situation through which Amy experienced? Extremis is a medical term that describes near-death state. And the ongoing resuscitation shows a multiple effort to keep her alive. Apparently, Amy's situation was so bad that she was slipping in and out of death. How fortunate we were that Dr. Wales was skilled enough to quickly analyze the situation and respond appropriately where so many of his colleagues had failed.

The legal updates that Amy and I received from our attorneys over the months of Amy's effort to recover come by mail or through phone conversations. The updates are not always positive and they usually added stress to our lives, which were already stretched to its limits with disruption and financial challenges. Some of the developments were so grim that I often found myself hiding them from Amy, who responded to negative developments much more emotionally than I. Even *Blue Cross Blue Shield*, the insurance company under which Amy was covered during the botched surgery, contacted us via letter to inform us of their interest in reclaiming their lost funds since we were holding a third party liable for Amy's extra medical expenses. The letter indicated that they were interested in recovering their financial loss only if we were able to get a financial judgment in our favor; but if no settlement monies are obtained, then BCBS would not hold us liable for any of the additional expenses paid out for Amy's medical care.

All the developments of our malpractice lawsuit promise one certainty: the case will be pursued, but the defendants will not admit to anything out of the ordinary. They will attempt to place blame upon Amy for the injuries she sustained, even while she was unconscious and totally under the care of the physicians treating her. They will avoid looking at facts that Amy's health before the surgery was optimal for anyone her gender, age, and physical size. The fact that Amy never used any tobacco products, no illegal drugs of any kind or any alcoholic beverages will mean little to the defense. It only matters to the defense if she had been a user or abuser of any of these substances. In fact, the defense will only focus in on variables which build their defense or diminish our case.

Amy and I grew closer through this ordeal, even though I learned she had private concerns of my leaving her because of her injury-causing inability to function in several areas and perform basic household chores that most wives do for their husbands and households. She expressed these concerns to her mother, who eventually told me about them. But leaving Amy was never an option for me. The thought had never even crossed my mind. In fact, I was resolved to see her through this, because this was the first test of a marriage less than a year old. I felt that if we could weather this storm together, then any others that would surface throughout our marriage would pale in comparison. My commitment to her would result in my greatest blessing yet.

CHAPTER 14

Medical Malpractice

In 1999 the Institute of Medicine announced that as many as 98,000 Americans die every year from medical errors. Shocking as that revelation was, now it seems the estimate may have been low. A new study due out this week finds that the number of preventable patient deaths in hospitals is actually twice as high. According to Health Grades, the health-care-rating organization that conducted the study, needless deaths averaged 195,000 a year in 2000, 2001 and 2002. "That's the equivalent of 390 jumbo jets full of people dying each year," says Dr. Samantha Collier, Vice President of Medical Affairs.

Anne Underwood, *Newsweek Columnist,*
August 2nd, 2004 issue

I need to begin this segment of the book by making a statement on my earnest belief about medical malpractice contests: nobody wins in a medical malpractice lawsuit, no matter what the outcome.

Whenever there is a complaint of medical injury, either someone has been terribly injured or a serious charge has been made against the professional ability of a medical practitioner. In both cases, someone is the victim and the ramification of such a charge is unalterable. In a medical malpractice claim, someone has suffered loss and as the litigation process matures, someone is going to lose again. Even if the medical practitioner manages to escape liability, the practitioner's professional record is severely tainted.

The topic of medical malpractice stirs different responses from different people. When discussing medical malpractice with mostly anyone in or associated with the medical profession, it is almost impossible not to draw some degree of defensiveness. After all, medical practitioners spend tens of thousands of dollars and years of their lives in education to become licensed to practice medicine. Physicians are understandably very protective of their profession.

Medical malpractice is the same thing as medical negligence, which is the same thing as medical injury. Each of these terms have been and will be used throughout this book. Attorneys also use all these terms, and they all mean the same thing. So, what exactly is medical malpractice? Medical malpractice occurs when a physician fails to properly treat a medical condition and the negligent act or omission is the cause of a new or aggravated injury to the patient. When a health care provider does something he is not supposed to do, or doesn't do something he is supposed to, resulting in a worsened condition or injury to the patient, then malpractice has occurred.

The physician cannot be responsible for the original underlying medical problem. The negligence in medical malpractice cases can occur in a variety of situations, including but not limited to:

- A delay or failure in diagnosing a disease

- Failure to gain the informed consent of the patient for an operation or surgical procedure

- A surgical or anesthesia related mishap during an operative procedure

- A physician who has made the correct diagnosis, but fails to properly treat the patient's ailment

- Misuse of prescription drugs, medical devices, or an implant

Generally, to prove malpractice, plaintiffs need to have the *four Ds* of medical negligence. These four are:

Duty of Care – A doctor's duty to care for their patient, requiring adherence to a standard of reasonable care while performing any acts that could foreseeably harm others.

Dereliction of Duty – Whenever doctors fail to maintain the agreed-upon relationship with a patient or overstep their boundaries.

Direct Causation – The process of determining whether a physician's actions were the direct result of harm towards the patient.

Damages – Demonstrative loss or harm that has a quantifiable value such that a monetary payment can be made.

The protectiveness physicians have over their profession can often be a gray area where professional duty overlaps into questionable practices of personal obligation. Doctors who protect bad doctors by withholding critical testimony in medical malpractice cases undoubtedly taint the profession. The medical profession has certainly lost some of its luster over the past few decades. With ever-growing HMO's seemingly prioritizing dollars over health care needs, rising medical malpractice insurance costs and increasing negligence complaints against doctors and hospitals, the professional arena of doctors has become one more of survival and less of prestige.

Since the early 1990's, there have been countless individual claims of medical injury, many of which were tried unsuccessfully. Some in the medical profession and political arena argue that the majority of these medical malpractice lawsuits are frivolous cases filed by dishonest people all for the purpose of "striking it rich." This argument is the preferred haven for those who take the position against malpractice lawsuits. The argument sounds like a decent one and may even make sense to some degree, but it simply does not parallel with the facts.

It is agreeable that there are plenty of frivolous lawsuits in our court system, many of them quite ridiculous. Ever hear of the lawsuit brought by the woman who successfully sued McDonald's to the tune of over $1 million, only because she spilled hot coffee on herself? It's insane to think that our society cannot hold one woman accountable for her own clumsiness; and it's sad to think that McDonald's can be held liable for serving hot, fresh coffee to its customers. It is also not a stretch to think that outrageous verdicts like this one could open the floodgates to more, frivolous lawsuits.

But while there are plenty of frivolous lawsuits to go around, the argument that most of these are *medical malpractice* lawsuits is an argument that doesn't parallel with the facts. Those who oppose medical malpractice lawsuits often hold the position that most malpractice cases are frivolous because they know that all medical malpractice or medical injury lawsuits are brought *only* for monetary damages. Like any personal injury lawsuit, a medical malpractice case is for monetary damages, *not* for punishment to the doctor, *not* for restricting or removing his license to practice medicine, and *not* to prevent similar acts from happening again.

To the surprise of the American Medical Association and other medical groups, who have long contended that laws regarding the liability of health care professionals are too liberal and thus require tort reform, the *New England Journal of Medicine* reported that a Harvard study found that the current legal system already successfully sifts out frivolous claims against health care professionals.

The study was apparently conducted by the Harvard School of Public Health and the Women's Hospital in Boston, which found that 90% of all claims against health care professionals involved a severe injury; 26% of those resulted in death and 80% in disability. The study reported that 63% of the injuries were due to the negligence of a medical professional and that the vast majority of those claims the claims thought to be without merit did not result in compensation.

This study seems to validate what plaintiff and defense lawyers have known for a long time; that tort reform is a response to a campaign of misinformation by not only doctors and their professional organizations, but also by insurance companies that give preference to insurance company profits over the rights of health care professionals to affordable malpractice insurance and the rights of those patients injured by health care practitioners.

It doesn't surprise me that those opposing medical malpractice lawsuits do not perform their own research to support their beliefs regarding malpractice litigation. The evidential facts do not parallel with their erroneous beliefs, which are often used in a manner that could harm other people by limiting awards to those severely injured, as well as those already injured by medical negligence.

Can't the case be made that doctors aren't doing enough to rid their profession of the *bad doctors* who cause most of the malpractice claims? If doctors don't do enough to improve their profession by getting rid of the bad doctors, is it surprising that they won't do enough to verify the claims about the sources for high insurance premiums?

When a medical injury occurs, the severity of the injury is a variable. Sometimes an injury can result in a lifelong impact upon the victim, such as the wrong limb being amputated, limited use of a limb due to nerve damage from a surgery, or a medical malpractice error resulting in death. In such cases, no amount of money can bring full restitution.

The financial aspect of medical lawsuits is a valid concern to both the health care practitioner and the victim. The argument about financial compensation has always been about how much; obviously there are two sides of the issue: those of the physician/hospital/insurance company's side and those of the plaintiff, or injured party.

Victims of medical malpractice indeed deserve to be financially compensated for their loss. While no amount of money can ever correct the damage that has been done, it can help buffer the loss by eliminating related or unrelated financial strain to the victim and his family. In circumstances where the injured party will require ongoing medical care due to the injury, a financial reward assists them in being able to continue being treated.

Existing laws do not provide for "getting even" with the physician. There are other means for an injured patient to let it be known that the physician acted improperly. Such doctors can be reported to their local County Medical Societies, their State Board of Medical Examiners, their specialty organization, and to the hospital administrator where the event occurred. Under such circumstances, the doctor will be scrutinized, may be found guilty of improper behavior and corrected, but this doesn't result in a financial award to the injured patient.

Currently, only about 30% of all medical malpractice cases are successfully litigated. In our state, it's only 18% - less than a 1 in 5 success rate. Yet, doctors in our state are orchestrated in their campaign to limit malpractice litigation. As I am writing this, I am staring at a color postcard mailer from the State Physicians Alliance which claims, "Doctors are leaving (our state)". Also included on this card are bullet points claiming:

- Your doctor could be forced to relocate or retire

- "Defensive" medicine forces your monthly medical insurance premiums higher

- Frivolous lawsuits have created skyrocketing insurance costs

- Contact your State Senator and the governor

Amazing that even in a state where only 18% of medical malpractice cases are won by the plaintiff, doctors *still* complain that they aren't being treated fairly by the state's legal system. And isn't it rather interesting that it says a physician practicing "defensive" medicine can transfer the higher costs of doing so onto you through higher medical insurance premiums? Isn't this what happens in every other industry in America? Isn't it true that in a free-market system, when the costs of conducting business increases, so does the goods and services to accommodate higher operating expenses? While I appreciate their concern, I must address some of the points the State Physicians Alliance raises.

First, the level of difficulty in trying and winning medical malpractice cases forces most law firms to meticulously scrutinize these cases *before* accepting a case and filing the appropriate petition with the court. Any medical malpractice lawsuit requires that the suing party prove all the necessary parts of the case. It must be shown that the doctor had a duty to his patient which was breached, wherein he/she acted inappropriately. It must also be shown that the erroneous decision and/or action of the doctor or the appropriate action the doctor *failed* to perform resulted in some permanent harm. It must further be developed that the negligence by the physician predictably would cause an injury and that such injury was preventable by appropriate reasonable medical care of an appropriate quality not provided. A trial lawyer knows that each of these tests must be satisfied and will evaluate whether they can be successfully evidenced before committing to filing the petition.

Secondly, the burden of proof will always rest with the plaintiff and the success rate is already stacked against the plaintiff; the difficulty of the plaintiff winning a malpractice lawsuit becomes sort of a self-deterrent mechanism for attorneys pursuing frivolous malpractice claims. Most of today's laws addressing malpractice litigation already favor doctors and health care practitioners; and so, this is yet another hurdle to be considered before an attorney or law firm will take the case. But I will say that even if there are attorneys who advance frivolous medical malpractice lawsuits into the courts, then they are really no different than doctors who practice substandard medicine. They hurt their profession and make it difficult for the good professionals who share their vocation.

Third, is it frivolous lawsuits that have created skyrocketing insurance costs or questionable medical care? Or is it possible that many of those lawsuits against doctors weren't frivolous at all, but just labeled so by the medical community because they failed in court? The truth is, to those involved in the medical community, *every* malpractice complaint is considered frivolous – no matter what the evidential facts are.

Board-certified surgeon, Dr. Ira E. Williams, comments, "The great increase in medical malpractice suits has not been caused by a 'litigious' society, rapacious attorneys, inadequate liability caps or greedy patients. Negligent medical care happens, and since almost no regulation of medical negligence occurs within the profession, the courts are the only recourse a harmed patient has."

While legislators focus on the frivolity of medical injury cases, these politicians fail to recognize the real, valid medical injury complaints and the impact *award cap legislation* will have on medical injury victims. It is my belief that an attempt to place a financial award limit on every medical malpractice case makes no distinction between the degrees of negligence, nor a distinction between the variable injuries unique to each medical malpractice complaint. A financial award cap on every malpractice claim treats *all* medical injury grievances the same, looping the strong, severe injury cases (those in the winning 30%) with the many other medical malpractice cases that are lost in court.

To better illustrate what I mean, let's imagine that an imposed federal tort law limits any medical malpractice damages to a maximum of $250,000, per incident – including both compensatory and punitive damages, but not including attorney legal fees. Now let's assume a situation where, during a cataract surgery, a 76-year-old male loses vision in one of his eyes due to the surgical mistake of the surgeon; the man has suffered a horrible loss but still has vision remaining in his second eye. In trial, it is determined by a jury that his surgeon's negligence caused the man's vision loss. The man is awarded the federally imposed maximum of $250,000.00. Now imagine another situation where a young 8-year-old girl suffers an injury during surgery resulting in irreversible cerebral palsy. It was discovered that her surgeon operated on her while under the influence of alcohol. A jury determines in trial that the surgeon was unquestionably negligent and the girl is awarded the federally imposed maximum of $250,000, even though she will have to be cared for by her family throughout her remaining living years, enduring years of additional medical costs and no hope of ever fully recovering from the permanent brain damage.

It doesn't require a PhD in quantum physics to understand the difference in these two scenarios. An award cap limit does not consider the 8-year-old's lessened quality of life and her loss of lifelong income earning potential. Regardless, we're all made to believe that the best way to deal with malpractice lawsuits is to limit the awards the victims should receive. But the problem with an award cap limit is that it presupposes all medical malpractice cases are similar, when reality can clearly dictate that they aren't.

Here's a suggestion: how about we train doctors to be more caring, empathetic and considerate of their patient's needs. How about teaching them to listen better and talk to people the way they would like people to talk to them. How about we get them to learn that treating a patient is more than just about treating their illness? Rather than these doctors working faster trying to see more patients (and thereby creating a possible situation where malpractice can occur), let's get them to slow down and get to understand the human side of their patient. These are little differences that can go a long way, because patients will stay with doctors whom they like, trust and display an aptitude for clinical competence. Doctors who have a good relationship with their patients are less likely to have to practice defensive medicine and can really concentrate on the medical aspects of their profession.

I think the problem with many medical practitioners today is that they treat their patients as products or cases that need to be "handled" – much like that doctor, Gregory House, on the Fox Network former series, *House*. If you've ever watched, you'll notice how over-the-top the main character is, not excluding his rude, obnoxious and very self-centered demeanor; even though House is smart and uses unconventional methods to be the best at what he does – that is, diagnosing potentially fatal mystery illnesses in the nick of time – it is somehow supposed to be enough to make up for his many flaws. But the character's lack of compassion amplifies his lack of total care. Kudos to the actor, Hugh Laurie, for his near-perfect portrayal of the misanthropic character.

Who says that doctors can't be both competent and caring? Is it too much to ask? A doctor lacking in either is just opening themselves up to trouble in the event the doctor severely messes up on the competence side, because despite what many so-called experts would have us believe, there are *not* a lot of people out there just wringing their hands waiting for a perfect opportunity to sue. I personally know that where there are patients who like and appreciate their doctors, tremendous latitude will be given if a medical error or injury happens. (Amy and I liked and trusted Dr. Keel, and because of this, gave tremendous leeway involving prior incidents with the doctor before the obvious botched surgery of March 7th.) But if the doctor is a jerk and deals with his/her patient in a less-than-caring manner, then these physicians should not expect much forgiveness if a medical injury occurs.

Doctors are resolute to claim that malpractice lawsuits force them to practice defensive medicine. What this means is, the doctor will order medical tests, procedures, or consultations of doubtful clinical value to protect themselves from a possible malpractice lawsuit. Personally, I don't think this is such a bad idea if it forces doctors to practice with more consistency. But the problem with the doctors' argument on medical malpractice arises in two areas: The first problem is more billable services to the patient's insurance company and the second problem is listening to many doctors whine about it. Should it really be the doctor's concern that a patient's insurance is being billed more for diagnostic tests or for "questionably necessary" medical devices at discharge? Remember how the vascular surgeon balked at the idea of discharging Amy with a walker? Was he correct in doing this? Was he truly concerned about his patient? Or was he trying to impose some personal philosophy on a patient who had absolutely nothing to do with it? If the insurance company doesn't raise a stink about it, then why should the doctor? Wouldn't the doctor be better served worrying more about his own malpractice insurance rather than the patient's medical insurance? In my opinion, defensive medicine might be a necessary evil if it results in fewer medical errors, particularly against arrogant doctors like this vascular surgeon prick.

I would even go so far as to recommend that patients become defensive in their own approach to medical treatment, and here's why: A doctor practicing defensively is doing so on the premise that he's going to get sued if a medical error occurs, even though he doesn't know this will happen. As a patient, you can rest assured that if a medical error does occur, the offending doctor will act tactically to cover his tracks and thwart discovery, and this almost always happens. So why wouldn't you want to take precautions against your treating physician if he's already taking them against you? Be mindful of your treatment and the services your doctor provides, listen carefully to what he tells you, ask plenty of questions, and regularly obtain copies of your medical records. Maybe the doctor will sense your thoroughness and begin to treat you better than just a regular patient; the doctor may even begin to treat you as well as a colleague, friend or family member. Who knows – the doctor may even see to it that he never keeps you waiting 20 minutes past your appointment time.

CHAPTER 15

The Process of a Medical Malpractice Lawsuit

A medical malpractice case is the most difficult an attorney will ever manage. They are extremely time consuming and quite expensive. It is estimated that the average medical malpractice lawsuit costs $20,000 to $40,000 actual out-of-pocket cost from the time a complaint is filed until a jury reaches its decision. This does not include the cost of an appeal should that become necessary. Substantial verdicts by a jury for an injured patient against a health care provider are indeed appealed. So, it is obvious that lawyers will not want to take on medical malpractice cases unless there are severe and substantial injuries or a wrongful death of an individual who was a wage earner and had dependents. Just the initial evaluation of a medical injury case alone – the medical records and the determination of whether such a case can expect to recover damages – frequently costs upwards towards $2000. In more complicated cases, costs for trial preparation and experts can exceed $100,000.

Any medical malpractice case that makes it to court scrutinizes the facts of the case and the quality of the evidence. The facts of a medical malpractice case will answer the two all-important questions: who was at fault, and what are the damages? Successful pursuit of a personal injury claim must involve a party responsible for the injury and damages (or losses) for which you can be compensated. The evidence of a medical malpractice case must support the facts, which must be proven in a court of law. What this means is medical malpractice cases are very reliant on the availability of detailed reports, witnesses, and physical evidence. All these components are necessary to have a medical malpractice case.

The process of litigating a medical malpractice case involves several steps:

1. Hire an attorney to conduct preliminary investigation

2. Lawsuit/Petition filed with the court

3. Collect medical records and other documents

4. Conduct pretrial discovery (interviews, interrogatories, production requests, depositions)

5. Expert Depositions

6. Mediation and settlement negotiation

7. Trial preparation (Pre-trial) and Trial

8. Appeals process

The first step in determining if malpractice has taken place is to consult an attorney. It is always the attorney's obligation to determine as quickly and efficiently as possible whether there is a viable, actionable case. This is so because medical malpractice cases are complex, expensive to pursue, have a high risk of no recovery, and often involve a client's "personal" attachment.

I recommend that your lawyer be *specialized* in pursuing malpractice cases, because even under the best of circumstances the opposing attorneys will vigorously defend their client(s) against you. It is rare for a health care provider to ever settle a malpractice complaint early. You should expect the doctor or hospital to hire a lawyer who specializes in defending medical malpractice claims and you should anticipate the defense would almost certainly pull out all stops to fight your claim. Many insurance companies and hospitals have their own attorneys as part of the regular staff, in salary paid positions. They exist solely for the purpose of giving these entities a legal consult advantage in a lawsuit.

Because the defense will use attorneys who are seasoned in fighting malpractice cases, you will need to hire attorneys who specialize in medical injury cases who can take the fight to them. When you employ any professional, and particularly in a medical malpractice matter, you'll want to inquire into the attorney's education, training, background, and experience. Ask other lawyers if you must, which is one indication of reputation. Specifically, you'll want to find out how many medical malpractice cases such a lawyer has reviewed, and how many depositions of medical experts he has taken, how many medical malpractice cases he has actually tried in a courtroom, and what his win-loss record is for these cases. This is a lot of information to inquire about in the short moments you have to select an attorney, but in the end it'll be worth it.

Be mindful that plaintiffs and defendants do not use the same kind of medical malpractice trial lawyer. As a rule, those who represent injured patients (the plaintiffs), do not work for insurance companies, and do not represent health care providers. The opposite is also true. There are many sources of references but a good one for injured patients is the Association of Trial Lawyers of America.

When you initially go to talk to an attorney about a malpractice complaint, you will want to have supporting documentation (i.e. medical records, doctor's notes, operative reports, etc.) with you. The attorney will want them, so it helps to be prepared. In talking with you, the attorney will generally attempt to answer two questions: 1) was someone negligent in providing medical care to you, and 2) what injury resulted directly from that negligent care? If after your interview the attorney determines there is evidence that these two questions are affirmative, he will consult an expert who will review and analyze the case information. If the expert agrees there is probable cause for negligence, the attorney will prepare and file a petition for lawsuit with the court. This triggers the defendants "being served" and their attorneys file Responsive Pleadings (or Grounds of Defense) to the lawsuit your attorney has filed.

Once an attorney decides to accept your case, you will more than likely enter into an agreement with the attorney in which the agreement sets forth the method of attorney compensation. Typically, the attorney agrees to advance all costs, only to be repaid costs in the event of recovery. This is called a contingency. On a contingency fee basis, the attorney would receive a percentage of the gross recovery; if no recovery is won, the client will suffer no economic loss.

The prompt collection of evidence can make a big difference in successfully proving your case. Every patient is 100% entitled to have all copies of his/her medical records. The patient's right to see each and every medical record about him or herself is absolute. Medical records consist of many more pages, comments and parts than is frequently given the patient at initial request. I have learned that whenever a patient requests medical records, and certainly when a lawyer does so, health care providers are immediately alerted of possible investigation into malpractice and will do whatever they legally can to stall and obstruct the patient from getting complete information.

I have also discovered that when requesting medical records, it helps to know *how* to ask for them. Be prepared to pay a stout fee for the medical record photocopies. When asking for medical records, particularly when you want them for evaluating possible medical malpractice, be sure to request a legible copy of each and every page of the medical record, including all notes written and dictated by physicians, consultants, nurses, and other health care providers. Do not omit any pages, items, reports, records, or dictated summaries even if they are unsigned and not yet proofread. Any such materials may be sent when completed or corrected or edited, but at this time all existing records should be sent. Include an itemized bill for all these services.

The collection of documents is only part of a larger process called *discovery*. Discovery is the process of obtaining pertinent facts, including documents and other evidence relevant to the case. The discovery process is perhaps the most laboring and time-consuming aspect of litigating a medical malpractice case because the facts aren't always easy to obtain. It certainly requires patience, plus a degree of voluntary cooperation from those close to the incident being investigated. Absent this cooperation, the plaintiff's legal team will have to spend much time and lots of money to find relevant evidence. Generally, in malpractice cases those individuals close to the incident will try to shield each other, locking arms to make it difficult for the plaintiff to build his or her case. Most of the discovery process happens before a trial begins, but in rare situations, discovery can take place in trial during cross examination – like what happens in just about every *Matlock* episode (sorry – I couldn't think of a more recent example). Pretrial discovery can be divided into three parts:

- Written discovery

- Depositions of the parties and witnesses

- Depositions of expert witnesses

In the Written phase of the litigation, each party sends to their adversary written questions called interrogatories, along with a written request to produce copies of documents relevant to the case (production requests). Interrogatories must be answered truthfully, in writing, and the parties must swear to their answers under penalty of perjury. Both sides must turn over any and all documents that it has regarding the case.

Depositions are under oath testimonies that are conducted outside of court – generally in a lawyer's conference room. Depositions provide an opportunity for the lawyers to find out beforehand what the other party and witnesses will say at trial. Depositions are recorded by a court reporter from which transcripts will be made. Lawyers use depositions to assess their adversary. What kind of person are they? What type of appearance do they make? Is the person believable? Will the jury like them? Questions like these are what the opposing counsel will be looking to answer when they depose party witnesses. It is customary that your attorney will practice deposition questions with you. This is to help you prepare for antagonistic questioning before the actual deposition takes place.

After written discovery is completed and transcripts received, they are forwarded to your attorney's experts to confirm and finalize their opinions regarding the case. Once this is completed, the expert name(s) and case assessment/conclusion is sent to the defense counsel. Arrangements are then made for the defense counsel to depose the plaintiff's expert(s). Like other primary testifying witnesses in the case, the experts will undergo a pre-deposition conference to make sure they are fully prepared, that they understand the facts of the case and what the issues are and that they understand what questions to expect. After the defense counsel has received the transcripts of the depositions of the plaintiff expert(s), they will disclose their expert(s) for the plaintiff's counsel to depose.

Most medical malpractice cases do not go to trial. The overwhelming majority of them settle, but of the medical malpractice cases that do make it to trial, most result in verdicts for the defense. The reason for this is that the insurance companies settle most of the cases they feel they are likely to lose. Usually, there are no serious discussions of settlement in medical malpractice cases until after the plaintiff's experts have been deposed. Even when a medical malpractice case goes to trial, some negotiations will usually have taken place beforehand.

When negotiations towards settlement are unsuccessful, the parties will agree to participate in either mediation or arbitration. Mediation is a form of negotiation where the attorneys and the clients agree on a neutral mediator, often a retired judge or experienced attorney, who will sit down with the parties and try to help them reach an agreement. Arbitration involves both sides agreeing on a neutral arbitrator who will actually decide the case with both sides agreeing to abide by that decision. Also, agreements to arbitrate usually include a "high/low" agreement. A high/low agreement means the parties have agreed that no matter how much money the arbitrator awards the plaintiff, the defense will not have to pay any more than the agreed upon high amount. It also means that even if the arbitrator decides for the defense and awards the plaintiff no damages, the plaintiff still gets the agreed upon low amount. If you agree to mediation, check with your attorney to determine whether there is a high/low agreement involved.

If the defense does not make a fair offer, then the case is set for trial. The experts will be contacted to testify at a specific date and time at trial. Your attorney will have exhibits prepared along with visual aids. This is where all the preparation comes to a head. If your attorney prepared adequately, then everyone testifying as a witness for your team will be prepared. Your case will be made before a jury of individuals from the county where the medical injury occurred.

If a medical malpractice complaint is to be pursued, then time is always of the essence. Each state has a *statute of limitations*, or a time limit set by law, which creates a deadline for filing a lawsuit, although some states allow extensions or have exceptions to their time limits. A suit filed after the deadline will be thrown out. Every state has its own special requirements. In our state, the statute of limitations is two years or 24 months from the date of the implied injury. Because of the statute of limitations, starting the claim as soon as possible is beneficial to any case in which medical malpractice injury is suspected.

Medical malpractice lawsuits necessarily take at least two years from the time you decide to litigate until a jury reaches their initial verdict, if it goes to trial. That is probably optimistic. It is not unusual for three years to elapse. If a substantial verdict is obtained one must plan an extra year for resolution of the appellate process, which is the defendants' opportunity to appeal a case verdict. Cases do settle before and instead of trial. However, usually all the preliminary work must be performed, and a settlement may be reached shortly before trial begins. That is the most common scenario. However, all cases must be planned to go to/through trial. Any client or lawyer who plans that a case will be settled without trial is possibly weakening the case, diminishing its value, and making it a great deal easier for the defense.

Judges can play a role in the outcome of a medical malpractice trial. Judges are appointed from different legal backgrounds; while they are supposed to be impartial in applying the written letter of the law, they can at times slant in favor of the plaintiff or the defendant. This sometimes manifests in leniency towards one side over the other, or what the judge will allow in terms of testimony. Liberal judges tend to be more lenient toward the plaintiff's case whereas conservative judges tend to be more lenient toward the defense. This is not so much a matter of right or wrong as it is a matter of judicial philosophy.

If the case evidence is strong, then it really shouldn't matter what the judicial philosophy of the judge is. Clearly, attorneys have their preference on which judge they would have presiding over a case. Experienced attorneys will know if the judge hearing the case will allow them to present the case, or stifle it with procedural penalties, etc. Regardless, the best judges are the ones who are truly impartial.

CHAPTER 16

What if I'm a Victim of Medical Malpractice?

Once a plaintiff sues, there will be a vigorous defense and the doctors and defense lawyers will try to beat them on every issue, no matter how obvious the apparent negligence may appear. In fact, the defense will do everything they can to beat the plaintiff. Besides trying to show that there was no negligence, or no damage caused by the allegation, the defense may argue that something or someone else actually caused the injuries. They will attempt to show the plaintiff received good medical care and indeed call it exemplary medical care. They will argue that the plaintiff is entitled to no damages and anything that is wrong, even in cases where death has occurred, was caused by the illness or some unforeseen circumstance; certainly not by anything the physician or other health care provider did wrong. They will frequently attempt to blame the patient or third parties, which may or may not exist for anything that went wrong. A defense tactic that is often employed is to blame the patient for the problem. Blaming the patient takes many forms including arguing that the patient was too fat, too thin, had unusual internal anatomy, was a smoker, a drinker, a drug abuser, did not take his medicine, failed to tell the doctor something he should have, or failed to come back as instructed. In the case of my wife's injuries, soon afterwards Dr. Keel asserted that Amy was too thin, had unusual internal anatomy, even blamed the error on a malfunctioning medical device (trocar).

Additionally, any part of the patient's background will be called into question, such as drinking habits, smoking, drugs, narcotics, marital infidelity, divorces, abortions, and even unimportant missed appointments. These defenses are an attempt to put the patient on trial instead of the doctor, or at least to try to get the jury to divide responsibility between the patient and the health care provider. Shameful, I know – but it is guaranteed to occur during the defense.

Obviously, medical malpractice litigation is serious business. So serious, in fact, that in effort to assist doctors and the attorneys who defend them, the *Physicians Malpractice Insurance Company* (PMICO is the malpractice insurer of most physicians in our state) posted the following information on their website regarding preparing for depositions:

Some Helpful Hints for Depositions – for doctors & medical staff insured by PMICO:

One of the most important aspects of successfully defending a medical malpractice action relates to the actual taking of the defendants' deposition. How well prepared you are and indeed how you conduct yourself at the deposition can play a critical role in the outcome of the lawsuit. Therefore, understanding what a deposition is about and how to adequately prepare become extremely important.

Your attorney will no doubt brief you prior to the actual taking of your deposition. You should plan to spend enough time at this briefing, (as uninterrupted as possible), in order to go over all aspects of the case and the likely areas of inquiry. We cannot substitute that preparation with this written document; however, we do recommend you review this document for some basic information.

THE DEPOSITION

An oral deposition is your testimony given before a court reporter, usually only with you and respective attorneys present. Depositions are important in the preparation of a case for trial. A deposition serves five basic functions:

    1.   It is used for the discovery of facts in the particular case.

    2.   It freezes your testimony at a given point in time and can be used for what is called impeachment if you deviate from it later. You can be asked the identical

questions again at the trial. If the answers you give at the trial are different from the ones you gave in the deposition, the variances could be used to challenge your credibility concerning all of your testimony.

3.   The probing and searching in a deposition are used to discover additional witnesses and to enable both sides to obtain depositions from them also.

4.   The collected testimony is used to narrow the issues in the particular case.

5.   The testimony given allows the attorneys to develop the facts and evaluate the merits of the case and, if possible, attempt to settle the case out of court.

RULES REGARDING DEPOSITION

To prepare you for the taking of your testimony for a deposition, your attorney would probably brief you on the following points:

1.   Review all of your files and the facts of the case and recount any procedures in question for the particular case. Giving deposition as a defendant is different than being called as an expert witness. The pressure is usually greater and attention to fine detail is greater.

2.   Always tell the truth. This is the self-preservation rule for a witness. Don't try to cover a mistake. If you make an error, simply state you were mistaken and correct your statement.

3.   Take time, go slow, and think before you speak. Listen attentively to the question and think a few moments to formulate your answer. Ponder the question and frame the proper response in your mind before speaking.

4.   Answer only the particular question you are asked and nothing more. Do not volunteer any additional information. Never give in to a compulsion to say more. If you don't understand the question precisely, don't attempt to rephrase it.

5.   Do not ever guess. If you don't know, say so. If you don't recall, say so. If the question involves a complicated procedure, or chain of events, summarize it if at

all possible. The more detail you try to cover in your answer, the more likely you will make an error in recall.

6.   Never characterize your testimony. For example, never say "in all candor," "honestly," or "I'm doing the best I can."

7.   Try to always avoid the use of absolute pronouncements, such as "I never" or "I always," and other such statements.

8.   As mentioned, your deposition is being used to freeze your testimony and the examiner will often ask, "Is that all there is?" You need to think carefully and clearly before replying that it is.

9.   If a document is an exhibit at the time of deposition, and you are asked a question about that document, you should take the time to thoroughly examine the document before answering any questions about it.

10.   Do not let the examiner put words in your mouth. Do not accept his characterization of time, distance, personalities, events and similar things. Restate it again in your original, or previous, words.

11.   Pay particular attention to the introductory clauses preceding the body of a question. These are the so-called "leading questions" which are often preceded by statements that are either half-truths or contain facts the examiner knows not to be true. He is trying to get you into a set of facts, some yours and some his, and commit you to a yes or no answer for the entire set.

12.   If you are caught in an inconsistency in a deposition, don't collapse. What happens next will usually depend on what the next question is and your attorney will have an opportunity to rehabilitate you either later in the deposition or at the trial stage.

13.   Do not accept the examiner's summary of your prior testimony. Often the examiner will ask a series of questions, sometimes in chronological order, stopping and summarizing and trying to commit you to a yes or no answer by suddenly saying, "Is that correct?" or "Would you say that is an accurate statement?" Simply reply that your previous statements were accurate and you stand on your testimony.

14.   Do not expand on an answer to a question when you feel it is complete. Often the examiner will continue to stare at you as if he expects more until you feel obligated to tell more.

15.   Never volunteer to supply any documents or other evidence. Leave that to your attorney.

16.   When an objection is made by your attorney to a particular phrase or question, listen to the objection very carefully. Often your attorney's objection will be worded to give you an insight into the problem he sees in the question and will help you, or hint how you can best answer the question.

17.   Never express anger or try to argue with the examiner. Your attorney should handle any unpleasantness. Testify in a calm, confident manner and do not attempt levity or suggest even the mildest obscenity.

18.   When things are said "off the record," be extremely cautious. Be sure that nothing you say can be overheard by the plaintiff's attorney, or any of his party, because even though the court recorder is not putting it down, the attorney could use it against you later.

19.   Do not attempt to educate the attorney if he seems confused or unable to comprehend a term or procedure you have mentioned. Many times, this is a trap to get you to expand your information.

20.   Everyone will make a mistake in giving testimony whether for a deposition or at a trial. Don't panic or get upset, there will be an opportunity to correct it later.

21.   Do not hesitate to ask your attorney about anything you do not understand. When you do not feel right about a question, or a procedure, you may ask at any time to consult privately with your attorney. It is far better to delay and be sure before answering.

22.   Wait until the complete question is asked. Many times, the last few words of a question change its meaning completely. Consequently, wait until the entire question is asked before attempting to answer.

23.   Always think through your answer. Time does not show in the transcript of a deposition, and it will not be apparent unless it is a videotape deposition. Therefore, if you need a minute or two or more to think through your answer, take it.

24.   When you are looking for something in the records while your deposition is being taken, do not speak. At this time it is very easy to be thinking out loud and not really be intending to say anything. However, the court reporter is taking down every word that is said and you may inadvertently say something at this particular time that you really did not intend to.

25.   It is much better to refer to the medical record and get the exact quotation than to take a dogmatic stand and be incorrect.

26.   Be very careful in acknowledging any Individual or book as an "authority." Medicine regards authorities differently than does the law. In law, if you regard any book or any doctor as an authority, you almost endorse anything that he has ever said, written, or will say or write. In actuality, books and articles do not treat patients, doctors do. Consequently, the best "authority" is the well-trained physician that is present, seeing the patient and taking care of the patient.

27.   (Our state) law recognizes community standards. In other words, the actual test in any given case is (1) what are the standards of the community? And (2) was there a violation of those standards? The plaintiff's attorney will probably approach this by asking if the practice of medicine in this community is of as high a standard as anywhere in the United States. It really is not a question of high standards, but of the practice utilized in a given community. He may also try to circumvent community standards by asking if the tests that are used for board certification are the same throughout the United States. Obviously they are, but that still does not have anything to do with peculiar or different practices in a given community. If you have practiced only in this community, you should not speculate on standards elsewhere.

This information was pulled directly from the malpractice insurer's website. I included this information to convey how thoroughly the defendant covers its bases. They will be highly prepared, and you must be too.

When the fight begins, a plaintiff needs to realize that it is a war between them and defense. The defense will go to the extent of what the law allows to fight the plaintiff's claim. To them, it doesn't matter that the patient was injured; it doesn't matter how or why; it doesn't matter if they lost a limb or partial use of it; it doesn't matter that they've been scarred and disfigured for life; it doesn't matter how much pain they went through or how much they've suffered; it doesn't matter that they almost died; it doesn't even matter to them if they did die, because it is a war. This war transcends their ability to extend human compassion to the plaintiff, because their sole job is to defend their client. The defense cannot be concerned with the plaintiff's loss, pain or suffering, because they exist only to get the plaintiff's case dismissed or at least limit the amount of damages their client may suffer as a result of the plaintiff's lawsuit.

Assuming that you are the plaintiff, through all of this the defense counsel will make you feel as though your complaint is without merit or justification. You will be led to feel guilty for taking action to protect your own interests. You will be challenged to determine whether your motives are genuine or whether you are a cash-seeking greedy leech. During these moments, it is helpful to remember that while the defense may question your integrity, *they* themselves don't work for free. Defending doctors is a big business, and theirs is a business that defense attorneys want to keep because it pays so well. And as ironic as it may seem, these defense attorneys need plaintiffs to sue their clients so they can remain employed. Also consider this: isn't it more likely than not that if any of these defense attorneys found themselves in your situation – that is, they or someone in their immediate family suffered trauma because of medical negligence – they would be inclined to file their own malpractice lawsuit?

In my personal experience, the defense looked thoroughly into our personal background, pulling our State Bureau of Investigation reports, requesting prior tax returns and required us to signed Medical Release Authorization forms for them to obtain unrelated medical records, and anything else they figured they could latch onto to possibly use against us to diminish our case and credibility. Fortunately, there were no negative issues in my or Amy's background to aid them – but there was one matter that surfaced with Amy's left knee, which she injured on a job many months *before* we were married.

The defense is being creative in trying to use this prior left knee injury in an effort to nullify the more recent left knee injury Amy sustained in the hospital. I will cover more on this in the *Building the Case: Larren vs. Defendants* portion of this book.

Always remember that once discovery gets underway it is possible that you will not hear from your attorney for weeks or even months. This doesn't mean your attorney hasn't been working for you. There is a lot of investigation, preparation and other things going on behind the scene, that does not require your direct involvement. Your attorney will contact you only when he needs to, and usually not before. While it is good to periodically get updates from your attorney – about every two months or so – I really wouldn't worry if you are not hearing from him every other day. Actually, if you are getting frequent calls from your attorney's office it might be a sign that he is relying more on you to provide key details about the case rather than finding those details through discovery. Also, it might be a sign that he has no other case work going on, which might be another negative sign; there could be a reason why he isn't busy.

The whole experience of a medical malpractice lawsuit can very well wear you down, so you must understand that the best thing you can do in the two to three (or four...or five) years it takes to litigate one is put it in the back of your daily life and *get on with living*. A malpractice lawsuit can bring a lot of anxiety, worry and can eat away at you if you let it. But if you have taken your time to hire an experienced lawyer with a reputable firm, then let them the worrying. Honestly, there's nothing you can do to advance a malpractice lawsuit without your attorney, so let him handle it; all of it – including the worrying.

Finally, attorneys are, by their very nature, cautious and legalistic, but they exist to conduct a legal service for you. Don't be ashamed to ask your attorney to clarify or re-explain something you didn't quite understand. Another thing: if you are concerned that your attorney isn't doing things your way, remember that *he* is the expert – not you. Ask questions if you must but trust his judgment. If after your attorney has begun work on your lawsuit and you find that you don't like the way he's doing things, NEVER fire him if you can absolutely avoid it. Doing so will minimize any compensation you might have coming. If the attorney has invested firm resources into your case, he is entitled to collect these monies when your case settles or reaches a verdict, even if he wasn't the attorney who represented you at mediation or during court.

CHAPTER 17

Damages & Compensatory Awards

"Damages" is a legal term for loss. It is money awarded to one party based on injury or loss caused by the other. There are many different types or categories of damages, and these categories can occasionally overlap, but for the purpose of medical malpractice, we will examine only two: compensatory and punitive.

Compensatory damages are those that cover actual injury or economic loss. Compensatory damages are intended to put the injured party in the position he/she was in prior to the injury. Compensatory damages typically include medical expenses, lost wages and the repair or replacement of property – also called "actual damages."

Punitive damages – sometimes called exemplary damages – are awarded over and above special and general damages to punish a losing party's willful or malicious misconduct.

As I mentioned before, medical injury lawsuits are brought *only* for money damages. Truly, there is no reason to litigate one except that a financial resolution is reached, because although the injury, pain and suffering can never be reversed by any amount of financial compensation, a large compensatory award can help offset a plaintiff's future medical expenses, loss of future income, loss of quality of life, etc. The legal conclusion of any medical negligence case is an award in the form of money damages. If a conclusion is a "$3 million verdict for the plaintiff, with $1.8 million of that being punitive damages", then it is understood that the remaining $1.2 million is for compensatory damages.

Many potential plaintiffs make the mistake of immediately thinking their case is worth many times more than it might be. This isn't because the plaintiff is trying to gain a ridiculous financial windfall from the injury. It is because these plaintiffs know first-hand how devastating the injury has impacted them in daily living. They personally know the details of how the injury impacted their life in a way that no other person could know. No one – not even your attorney – can appreciate the severity of the impact the injury placed on the plaintiff. The plaintiff knows intimately how it has interrupted life, and this is a reality that is extraordinarily tough to convey to a jury who just sees the "facts" presented before them by attorneys from both parties.

Still, no one should try to guess the value of a malpractice case. The value of a case generally depends on what a jury thinks is fair compensation for the injuries sustained. The jury is the final arbiter, and only in some occasional instances, the best. The true value of a medical injury case depends on many issues: the kind of malpractice, the nature of the injury, the severity of the injury and whether it is permanent, the believability and credibility of the witnesses, whether the jury likes the victim and the victim's family, whether the doctor is credible and believable or looks and acts like a liar or possibly someone who just doesn't care. Just as the plaintiff will be properly prepared to be a witness, instructed on how to behave and how to appear, so will all the health care providers for the defense be groomed, trained and practiced to win.

Since each malpractice case is as unique as the people who are involved in them, there is no point in trying to guesstimate how much any malpractice case is worth by trying to compare it to similar cases. There are just too many variables involved to guess accurately what a case is worth. My advice is to allow your attorney to work the case his way to get an award for maximum damages.

Informed consent cases by themselves generally do not win any compensation in medical malpractice lawsuit. Informed consent is a legal requirement where the doctor or other health care provider is required to get a patient's permission to perform a certain procedure. The patient must be told the essential risks, benefits, and alternatives of a procedure and accept those, sometimes in writing. If the patient is not told anything and a procedure is performed which ends up being harmful, this is the beginning basis for suing for failure to get the proper informed consent for the procedure. A result of this simple definition lays a big problem: further requirement is for the patient to credibly and believably state that if they knew the risk but were uninformed, they would have refused the procedure and not accepted treatment. There are very, very few times when this is believable. Therefore, most informed consent cases are usually coupled within other kinds of medical malpractice cases.

An experienced attorney will know exactly what kind of evidence and documentation is required to prove damages and maximize a plaintiff's recovery, but the amount of compensation the plaintiff is entitled to receive is entirely dependent upon the damages the attorney can prove. The calculation of these damages will take into account the plaintiff's medical bills, lost time from work, limitation on future employment, disfigurement, pain and suffering, rehabilitation time and expenses.

As Amy's husband, my attorneys informed me that although I wasn't the one who was injured, I have a compensatory damage claim for loss of spousal services and companionship. This means, as a result of the medical injury, Amy's function in our household was nonexistent during her recovery. The flipside to this is as she improves and continues to get better, my claim for loss diminishes.

There is no way to determine exactly the value of our case. It is quite possible – in spite of all the evidence – that we could end up with nothing for all the pain, suffering and mental anguish that Amy endured. While the thought of this doesn't sit well with me, the reality is that the tort laws of today are stacked against plaintiffs. These laws exist to discourage a trend of legal action against medical practitioners. In the effort to discourage the trend, the laws stack the odds against the injured party and instead make a victim out of the health care practitioner.

Obviously, damages are such an important part of any case litigated. Where malpractice negligence or intentional wrongdoing causes injury to another party, the degree and scope of the injury, negligence or wrongdoing is often in direct proportion to how much the injured party is compensated. Two good legal movies I can recommend are *Erin Brokovich* and *A Civil Action*. Neither of these movies is solely about medical malpractice, but they both offer a good insight into lawsuits, the discovery process, and how lawsuit cases are built and conducted.

While the information here provides only a basic look at damages in medical injury cases, a practicing trial attorney can more thoroughly explain the different types of damages and compensation for plaintiffs of medical negligence.

CHAPTER 18

Expert Witnesses, Standard of Care, and the Medical Code of Silence

When it comes to medical malpractice litigation and trial, both parties will have to present a testifying witness that qualifies as an *expert*. In the broadest definition, an expert is a person having special knowledge, training, or experience in the technical field of subject in a trial. An expert witness is permitted to state his/her opinion concerning technical matters even though he/she was not present at the event. Because an expert has special knowledge in a particular field, it entitles them to testify their opinion on the meaning of facts. Non-expert witnesses are only permitted to testify about facts they observed and not their opinions about these facts.

In a medical malpractice case, an expert witness is usually a physician that has medical training or experience in the same field as the defendant. Ideally, the expert will be a doctor currently practicing (or working) on a day-to-day basis in the field they will be testifying about. An expert who is retired from the field or one who only does research or writes journal articles isn't as credible as an expert who practices in the field.

For the plaintiff, it important that they enlist an expert witness that lives in or near the community or area where the injury occurred. This is true because of something called Standard of Care.

Standard of Care is a diagnostic treatment process that a practitioner should follow for a certain type of patient, illness, or clinical circumstance. In legal terms, standard of care is the level at which the average, prudent provider in a given community would practice. It also encompasses how similarly qualified practitioners would have managed the patient's care under the same or similar circumstances. Like all states, your state has a statute, case law, or jury instructions defining what the *standard of care* should be, how the proof of skill or reasonable treatment is to be presented, and whether it is to match local standards or national standards. Sometimes the standards between office and hospital-based physicians vary. Frequently there is a different standard set by law for emergency room physicians than for others. Failure to meet the standard is negligence and any damages resulting may be claimed in a lawsuit by the injured party. The problem is that the "standard" is often a subjective issue upon which reasonable people can differ.

All these are generally legislative differences. A health care provider is to do the right thing at the right time, in the right way for the right reason. The health care provider should anticipate a result and if such a result is not achieved, then inquire why that occurred and to make a correction if necessary. The standard of medical care required is *good* medical care. The defense prefers to look at what the *average* health care provider does under defined circumstances. Good medical care requires a proper response – not necessarily what the majority of people would do under such circumstances.

Still, a standard of care can vary from one part of the country versus another. Climate, social environment, and available resources are just some of several reasons contributing to a regional standard of care variation. Under similar circumstances, certain treatment practices followed in one area do not necessarily parallel to that of another hundreds of miles away. So an acceptable medical treatment practice in a southwestern state like Arizona can vary from a medical treatment practice in a New England state of the northeast. Because of this, any standard of care question has to be compared to what the *local* medical community accepts as a common treatment practice or response to a given patient, illness, or medical situation.

The plaintiff in a medical malpractice case must establish the appropriate standard of care and demonstrate that the standard of care was breached. This almost always creates a problem for the plaintiff because the foundation to establish this successfully rests on finding a doctor from the *same* community testifying as an expert witness that the defendant failed to follow a standard of care. This hurdle is a significant one to overcome because of a disappointing secret that exists within the medical community, and it wouldn't be an overstatement to call this secret a conspiracy.

Many of us have heard of *"the blue wall of silence"*, which is known as the unwillingness of law enforcement officials to testify against members in their own profession. There is a similar, unwritten but understood code of silence amongst those in the medical field. This code is virtually universal rather than confined to a single community, area or region of the country. The secret about which I'm referring is what I call the *Medical Code of Silence*.

The Medical Code of Silence is the reality in which doctors will not testify against other doctors. Our experience has taught us that doctors will not voluntarily speak out against other doctors and will avoid providing testimony against the same, even in cases where improper care or negligence is suspected. It is far easier for a doctor to remain silent than to become involved and possibly provide condemning testimony in a matter where their opinion can make a substantial difference in the outcome of a medical malpractice complaint.

If subpoenaed by the court, the summoned doctor may be evasive in cooperating with the plaintiff's counsel while answering questions that could harm a colleague caught up in a malpractice contest. There are reasons why this happens – one being that the subpoenaed doctor may realize that he/she might one day be involved with their own malpractice fight. A doctor called to the stand against a local practicing physician will be evasive answering questions in court, in hopes that the ambiguity will in favor be returned should the doctor ever find him/herself in a similar situation.

Violating doctors, or doctors who break the Medical Code of Silence and willingly testify against other local doctors, are shunned, and blacklisted by the other practitioners within that local medical community in response to their violation. A doctor who violates the Medical Code of Silence is denied patient referrals from colleagues. This backlash is a direct negative impact on the violating doctor's practice and affects the doctor's ability to advance in their area of medicine. It limits the violating doctor's income and prestige.

Another reason doctors refuse to testify against each other is perhaps the most degrading insult projected toward a violating doctor. Breaking the Code will in effect exclude the violating doctor from professional recognition, social gatherings such as cocktail parties and other similar events. They are in a sense ostracized by their professional peers.

Although these mentioned reasons might seem severe enough to prevent a local doctor from serving as an expert witness for a plaintiff, there is still yet another reason doctors in a given community will not testify against others in the same.

I learned that in our state, most of the state's practicing physicians share a common malpractice insurance carrier. PMICO (Physician's Malpractice Insurance Company) covers a vast majority of the doctors in the state. If, by reasons of litigation, PMICO decides to raise its premiums, it does so across the board affecting all doctors insured by the carrier – regardless of if an individual practitioner has ever been accused of negligence. In other words, doctors who practice good medicine are penalized with higher malpractice premiums along with, and because of doctors who practice bad medicine.

An insurance carrier will share the cost of an increasing risk amongst all of the insureds (or the participants in coverage). This is also true for PMICO. Doctors in our state who choose not to testify in a case against another local doctor reap a backdoor economic benefit in making that choice. They realize that when a local doctor – any local doctor – is sued and that suit becomes a judgment in favor of the plaintiff, the possibility of their own malpractice insurance premium increasing is more probable. I suspect this situation also exists in other states.

Any or all these reasons can hinder a plaintiff's ability to locate a local expert witness for their case.

While there is little love between doctors and their defense attorneys, most doctors would rather testify in favor of a colleague than testify against. This has little to do with helping the defense attorney and everything to do with helping their colleague, their profession and ultimately, themselves. The consequences in doing so are minimal and it affirms to the local medical community that the doctor is a willing defender and protector of the "club". A doctor who testifies on behalf of a colleague as a defendant's expert witness doesn't risk much and volunteer free testimony without compensation. Defense attorneys have no trouble finding a local physician to aid them as expert witnesses in a medical malpractice suit.

Except in the rarest of incidents, a plaintiff must always rely on an out-of-state expert witness to help their case. This expert witness must be hired and compensated for their services. At the appropriate time, the plaintiff's chosen expert will travel to the local community hosting the trial. The plaintiff's expert witness will have to be compensated for travel, in addition to payment for time spent with the plaintiff's attorneys for discovery review, consultation phone time, and testimony in trial. Without explaining why the expert was paid, defense attorneys will point out to the jury during trial that the plaintiff's expert was paid, implying that the expert testimony of the plaintiff was "purchased." It is up to the plaintiff's counsel to educate the jury why the plaintiff's expert is paid and why the defendant's expert witness is not.

With qualifications of both expert witnesses equal, standard of care tilts qualification in favor of the defense's expert witness because the plaintiff's expert witness may not be able to overcome the stigma of being a non-local physician. The defense will always have an easier time explaining to a jury that a standard of care was not breached since the defendant's expert witness will most likely be a local physician practicing in the local community. The obvious question of whether a plaintiff's expert witness (who doesn't practice medicine in the local area) really knows the local standard of care is something that will enter a juror's mind. Couple this with the probability that the defense counsel will illustrate that the plaintiff's expert witness was paid to appear at trial as an expert, it is easy to see how a juror might intentionally or subconsciously conclude the expert witness of the plaintiff is less credible than that of the defense'.

In our personal malpractice case, Dr. Reysa, Amy's current gynecologist, was interviewed by our attorneys to feel out is position as a potential expert witness for our case. He was also interviewed by the defense counsel of Dr. Keel. Dr. Reysa informed our attorneys that his message to Dr. Keel's defense counsel was that they should save everyone the trouble of trial and simply compensate Amy for her injuries, because it was his opinion that Amy's injuries should have never occurred under any circumstance. While Dr. Reysa agrees that Amy's terrible injuries were avoidable and that negligence is suspect, our attorneys concluded that he would not be a credible expert witness for testimony because he doesn't and has never performed the laparoscopic procedure that Amy underwent. Dr. Reysa has a conservative approach to medicine, and he believes that often, less is more, claiming that many of the younger doctors are enamored with the new technologies available to them as they seek to use these tools before the medical need is clearly evident. Dr. Reysa said that the laparoscopic procedure performed on Amy was medically risky and why he doesn't perform them.

Dr. Reysa steered our attorneys to a doctor currently practicing in another part of the state. Dr. Reysa told our attorneys that this particular doctor that he recommended had "no friends" in the medical community. It was a promising lead, until our attorneys tracked this guy down and met with him about the possibility of becoming an expert witness. They discovered that this doctor had relocated to another part of the state as a sort of self-extradition and was attempting to establish a fresh start there. This doctor learned the hard way how quickly his profession can turn cannibalistic when the Code is broken. He did not want to spoil his new beginning by becoming involved in another malpractice case. The stakes were simply too high for him.

Because the effort to find an in-state doctor signing on as an expert in our malpractice case produced no takers, our attorneys had to settle on an expert witness who practices in an adjacent state, many miles away. In March of the following year, a solid full year later, Amy and I traveled to visit with Dr. Harren per the instruction of our attorneys. If our case went to trial, Dr. Harren can testify that he had the opportunity to examine Amy, though not as a treating physician. Dr. Harren reviewed Amy's medical records, identified several areas of negligence based on those records and will testify to such, if and when we get to trial. Also, Dr. Harren is being compensated for his services.

So high is the value of having a local expert witness to testify for a plaintiff that in some instances doctors will proactively project themselves into a situation where a malpractice suit is suspected. This is not some mere statement to elicit shock. Amy and I discovered that we were the possible victims of a doctor's interjection to subjectively impact our case during an emergency room visit in April, just a matter of weeks after Amy's March 7th botched surgery. It supplements my belief that doctors go out of their way to protect others in the profession, and we did not discover proof of this tactic until many months after the ER visit.

As I mentioned before, an April 1st emergency room visit revealed that Amy had sustained a fractured patella. The trigger sending us to the ER that day was Amy's complaining of constant, excruciating pain on the whole of her left leg. The attending physician was Dr. Elliott at the Lakeside North Medical Center.

At a deposition preparation meeting at our attorneys' office in the summer, four years following Amy's botched surgery, a portion of Amy's medical records were pulled from the very large case file. The records from this April 1st emergency room visit surfaced here for us to see for the first time since that visit. Our attorney asked us about the visit and read from the doctor's emergency room report:

"This is a 23-year-old white female who comes to the emergency department complaining of left knee pain. History is obtained from her husband. The patient herself is nonverbal during the observation. Despite my efforts I cannot get her to speak to me. Her husband speaks for her and is unconcerned for her lack of speech during this visit. She herself is nondistressed and agrees with her husband by shaking her head. He states that she suffered some medical misadventures at another hospital on 3/7/01 and since 3/14/01, while in the hospital, she has complained of pain at the proximal aspect of her left knee. She had x-rays at the other hospital and was told they were negative. She was given a walker to help her ambulance. She is running out of the Lortab 7.5 that she has been taking. She needs more. There is no new injury or new exacerbations of pain. The pain is at the same level that it has been. It is a severe constant pain. There is some difficulty determining exactly where it is tender or painful."

Our attorney was concerned about Dr. Elliott's wording of the emergency room report, commenting that the doctor's take and emphasis on my lack of concern for Amy's unwillingness to answer him was an effort to "weigh in" on what he suspected might be a malpractice case. Surely after examination, Dr. Elliott was aware that Amy had sustained injuries requiring at least one major surgery. The doctor admits in another area of the report that Amy "has healing surgical scars to the right chest wall, the abdomen and the inguinal region bilaterally." At first glance, when the report is read it appears that I am more interested in implicating the hospital rather than being concerned for my wife.

This, however, was totally untrue. Amy's health and comfort was my primary concern. My other concern was making sure the doctor had all the information he needed to properly treat her. Amy was not yet fully informed or aware of all that happened when she was in the hospital and could not appropriately answer the questions Dr. Elliott was asking. At this point, she was quite distrustful of doctors, which also contributed to her lack of communication with him.

What troubles me most about Dr. Elliott's emergency room report is the fact that in another part of the report he states Amy had "full range of motion without pain." The truth is he never tested her range of motion and if he *had* he would have discovered that she absolutely *did not* have full range of motion. At the time of this visit, no one knew about the femoral nerve damage affecting Amy's left leg. The nerve damage prevented her leg from functioning normally and severely limited her leg's strength, function, *and* range of motion. Why then is there a "full range of motion" record falsification? Did the doctor want to negatively influence a case he suspected existed against colleagues? He must have known that the medical records of this ER visit would be obtained if Amy and I had a medical malpractice case regarding her botched surgery.

Finally, before Amy and I were fortunate enough to find Dr. Reysa as her current treating gynecologist, we were first referred to another gynecologist by Dr. Sanders, the general practice medical doctor who coordinated Amy's post-discharge recovery. This is the same Dr. Sanders I mention before in earlier chapters. The OB/GYN to which Dr. Sanders referred Amy was Dr. Porter.

Dr. David Porter practices out of the Presbyterian Medical Center and is basically in charge of the entire obstetrics/gynecology unit there. He's touted in this area as the best in his field. His picture is on at least one billboard in our metropolitan city, and he has been featured in metro-area television commercials, where he speaks about the technology, experience and dedication his team brings to the women's health department at the Presbyterian Medical Center. Dr. Porter certainly comes off as a knowledgeable and honest professional who appears intelligent, focused and a community icon who is at the zenith of his profession. In fact, it was the reason Dr. Sanders recommended him. The appointment with Dr. Porter was initiated and arranged by Dr. Sanders' office. Prior to the appointment, his office was furnished with Amy's medical records and Dr. Sanders' own examination report beforehand.

In May, just two months after Amy's botched surgery, she had her first and only visit with Dr. Porter. Because of Amy's degraded physical state and ambulation problems, the only way for her to keep the appointment was for me to take her. We walked into Dr. Porter's office together upon our arrival and checked in with the receptionist. I did not accompany Amy during the examination. Comfortable in my knowledge that Dr. Porter already had the opportunity to view Amy's records, I was satisfied that he had all the information he needed to properly assess her, so I decided to stay in the waiting area while Amy went into the back.

After several minutes, Amy emerged from the back part of the office and began checking out with the receptionist. I remained seated, expecting Dr. Porter to come out and meet with me to discuss his findings, but he never did. As Amy made her way over to me, I noticed that her demeanor was uneasy and I asked her what was wrong. Amy answered, saying she did not want to see this doctor again because he appeared distant and intolerable. She was upset that he opined that her injuries were a *common and accepted* risk of having a laparoscopy procedure done. I thought this was quite egotistical, shallow and irresponsible of him to make such a comment while Amy's injuries were still being discovered. Nonetheless, Amy scolded me for not sitting in with her during the examination. Regardless, Amy's answer gave me the reason why this doctor never came out to talk with me or even introduce himself.

A day or two after Amy's appointment with Dr. Porter, our attorneys followed up with him to discuss his assessment of Amy's injuries and overall gynecological condition. Neither Amy or I, had talked with our attorneys about any specifics of her appointment with Dr. Porter prior to their meeting with him, but our attorneys were dismayed at Dr. Porter's casual attitude about Amy's injuries and speculation on how the injuries occurred. It was immediately apparent to them that they were getting nowhere with the doctor and our attorneys meeting with him ended far quicker than imagined. *But we were all blind sighted when we later discovered that Dr. Porter would serve as the expert witness for Dr. Keel, the primary defendant!*

Anger is too soft a word to describe my feelings when I learned of this. Knowing what I did about expert witnesses and *standard of care*, I felt that Dr. Porter's cooperation with our adversaries could be a catastrophic blow to our case.

Our attorney, Steve, in discussing his meeting with Dr. Porter, told me that he was not impressed with this doctor and said that under no circumstances would he ever let his own wife be treated by this man. He stressed this wasn't a retaliatory position based on the doctor's unwillingness to assist us; it was based solely on his conversation with Dr. Porter. Steve said that any doctor who could have such a calloused attitude to Amy's type of trauma has a deluded image of his patients and had lost a part of his humanity.

Imagine the irony of an attorney commenting about the lost humanity of a doctor. Dr. Anthony Fauci aside, jokes about attorneys are an accepted form of amusement while doctors are always presumed to be noble and flawless. It is only until one requires the services of an attorney that one entirely appreciates the service they provide. Another attorney (not affiliated with Steve or Frank) whom I consulted to review this book told me that this same Dr. Porter had treated his wife during her pregnancy. When the time came for his wife to give birth, the doctor stalled arriving at the hospital and instead tried to handle the situation over the phone. The doctor was in the middle of a golf game and apparently didn't want the emergency to interrupt him. Only until the attorney demanded the doctor's presence did he agree to suspend his golf game and appear at the hospital. The attorney's wife delivered within an hour and only 15 minutes of the doctor's arrival. Quite pathetic.

As our malpractice case continued to build against responsible parties, our attorneys later discovered that Dr. Keel had trained under Dr. Porter as a resident. She was his protégé. This being the case, what benefit would it ever serve Dr. Porter to testify against her? It wasn't enough for him to simply deny helping us. He was only satisfied when he had the opportunity to assist *opposing us*. It would seem that an apparent conflict of interest might keep Dr. Porter from opting to serve as an expert for our adversaries, but the fact that Dr. Keel trained under him won't stop him from testifying on her behalf. Is this unfair? Perhaps, but it is legal.

The situation we experienced with Dr. Elliott and Dr. Porter are impacting, negative developments that deserve being brought to light. I suspect that things like this happen all the time in medical malpractice cases, but the general population never knows about it. All we ever assume – because it's all we ever hear – is that the greedy plaintiffs are going after the victimized doctor. The physician charged with negligence is always given the benefit of the doubt – by the public, by the courts, legal system, and by other doctors.

For those who would argue that doctors are infallible, I offer this list of physicians as a counterargument: Dr. Death, Jack Kevorkian, like his World War II physician death camp counterparts who performed unspeakable deeds of evil at Auschwitz, are all fallible; Democratic National Committee Chairman, Dr. Howard Dean, is as fallible as any psychotic criminal in my opinion; Dr. Joycelyn Elders, the ex-Surgeon General appointed and fired by the incredibly fallible former President Bill Clinton, is certainly fallible herself; any doctor or medical scientist who accepts the deplorable act of destroying life, all in the name of embryonic stem-cell research, is fallible; any abortion doctor performing the intentional killing of unborn babies by literally dismembering them from the womb – all in the name of turning a profit, while at the same time denying the life and personhood qualities of an unborn child, even in our age of scientific enlightenment which proves otherwise, is certainly fallible; *any* doctor involved in a medical malpractice case is fallible. People are not infallible simply because they are doctors and based on the list above, they can be among the *worst* our society has to offer.

CHAPTER 19

Medical Injury and Malpractice Case Summaries

The following are actual cases involving real people. These cases were compiled from public access records and are all intentionally older cases to ensure that they all have already been legally concluded. Out of courtesy and respect for the victims, I have voluntarily altered the names of every individual plaintiff and as a vocational courtesy, I have voluntarily altered the names of individual defendants.

When reading through these, you will begin to see a pattern where the defendants 1) deny, 2) deflect, and 3) demean.

The first response is for the practitioner to deny aspects of the injury, whether its scope, depth, or denial that there is any injury at all – as if the patient is faking injury or perhaps not knowledgeable enough to ascertain whether they have an injury or not. In our malpractice situation, it was rather obvious that Amy suffered injury, but even so, subsequent doctors began to question the sincerity of Amy's discomfort (degree of pain) and the denial of other injuries – such as the pain in her fractured left patella. They wanted others to believe this discomfort was somehow mentally manifested.

If it is obvious or determined that an injury did occur, the second response is for the practitioner to deflect responsibility. In the case of the doctor responsible for Amy's initial injury, she blamed the trocar instrument, she blamed Amy's petite size and she also blamed Amy's physiology as being different than standard human physiology.

Lastly, the practitioner along with the practitioner's defense will attempt to demean the victims of a medical malpractice claim. To demean someone is to degrade or put down a person's character, status or reputation to minimize the seriousness of a matter. Again, while some of the doctors were credible and professional, too many of the doctors opined disparagingly about Amy and me – without any proof or evidence to give such adverse commentary – inserting themselves into a matter which they had no complete knowledge. They are motivated to protect a colleague, protect a profession, or to negatively hurt the credibility of our case or us as individuals. Where is the professionalism in this?

The chosen cases, tragic as they are, all resulted in some compensatory award for the victims – but keep in mind that in all of these cases, real damage had been done, up to and including death. And for the ones shown in this chapter of the book, there are far many more that do not reward adequately in light of the injury. Many medical malpractice claims never advance to trial if some pre-negotiated settlement is reached, which may or may not be sufficient for the aftermath of injury. In many cases, the plaintiffs end up with only 40 – 60% less of the awarded amount, the difference of which goes to the plaintiff legal team. In other cases, the state laws reduce or limit the jury awarded amount based on the tort laws that exists within the state where the injury occurred.

There are so many variables that need to be considered in medical malpractice cases, that from the onset, plaintiffs will face a difficult uphill battle. Keep this in mind as you read through these horrific medical malpractice cases.

Case Name: **Tim Veal vs. Dr. Dana Sconce**
Date: 12/16/02
Case Number: 00-CV-1450G
Court: Superior Court, Suffolk County, Massachusetts

Case Synopsis: This was a medical malpractice action in which it was alleged that the Defendant, Dr. Dana Sconce, was negligent in performance of a routine urological procedure. On November 16, 1998, Dr. Sconce performed a cystoscopy on Plaintiff, 79-year-old Tim Veal, to relieve a urinary stricture. When she was unable to find a urinary passage and opened the stricture during the cystoscopy, she attempted a percutaneous procedure to drain the bladder by inserting a trocar into the bladder. When this also proved unsuccessful, Defendant performed an open procedure to insert a catheter into the bladder through a supra pubic puncture. Another procedure was performed later the same day to check the potency of the catheter and insert a drain in the retroperitoneal cavity. Starting within an hour of the first surgery and continuing in the days that followed, Plaintiff's kidneys shut down, his abdomen became distended and he developed an ileus, among other symptoms of necrotizing fasciitis that went undiagnosed until the fifth day postoperatively. At that time, he was operated on to repair the necrotic tissue, which included his rectal sheath, oblique muscles, left testicle and testicular cord. Many more operations were necessary to resect additional necrotic tissue, complete a colostomy and reconstruct the abdominal wall.

Plaintiff alleged that Dr. Sconce punctured Mr. Veal's sigmoid colon during the initial insertion of the trocar, and the colonic contents caused the infection in the peritoneum. Plaintiff argued that Dr. Sconce was negligent in attempting to insert the trocar into a bladder that was not full and by failing to explore beyond the peritoneum when a portion of it was seen torn and bleeding during the second surgery on November 16, 1998. Lastly, it was argued that the Defendant was negligent for failing to diagnose the severe abdominal sepsis, peritonitis and necrotizing fasciitis at an earlier stage.

Defendant claimed that she did not puncture the sigmoid colon and the compromise of the colon wall was attributable to a diverticulum that became inflamed and burst on the fourth or fifth post-operative day. The records and the findings of the subsequent treating surgeon supported this position. Defendant also relied on the fact that several other specialists were involved in Mr. Veal's post-operative care and none of them diagnosed the sepsis or recommended an exploratory laparotomy.

The jury received the case at approximately 12:45 p.m. on December 10, 2002. At 4:00 p.m., the jury retired from deliberations for the day. Deliberations continued at 9:15 a.m. on December 11, 2002, and the jury returned a verdict of $7,143,561.30 at about 12:40 p.m. that same day. The verdict was comprised of $378,561.30 in past medical expenses, $5,000,000 in past pain and suffering and $1,765,000 in future pain and suffering. Over two million dollars of interest has accrued to date bringing the judgment to approximately $9,500,000. The only settlement offer was $300,000 communicated approximately two hours before the jury returned its verdict.

Conclusion:

Plaintiff's verdict for $7 million. Approximately $9,500,000 when interest is added.

Case Name:	**Estate of Yannis Creek and Elaine Whetmore vs. Dr. Ben Q. Swank and Massachusetts General Hospital**
Date:	10/15/99
Case Number:	97CV12134
Court:	United States District Court for the District of Massachusetts

Case Synopsis: Yannis Creek, age 35, and Elaine Whetmore, age 39, were diagnosed with glioblastoma, an invariably fatal form of brain tumor. They were both treated by Dr. Swank with boron neutron capture therapy, which was experimental, in which their brains were exposed to a beam of radiation. Plaintiffs claimed that the procedure caused massive brain damage and premature death, and that they did not learn what happened to their family members until the mid-1990s. Defendants denied wrongdoing.

Conclusion:

Plaintiffs' verdict for $8 million including $5 million in punitive damages.

Case Name: **Gardner vs. Galen Hospital of Texas**
Date: 3/12/99
Case Number: E-55812
Court: Superior Court, Fulton County, Georgia

Case Synopsis: Gardner, age 19, sustained a back injury and was taken by ambulance to Defendant hospital where she was assessed by an LPN. Despite complaints of severe back pain radiating into her lower extremities she was not treated as an emergency case and was removed from the back board upon which she had been transported to the hospital without a doctor's order. She was then transferred to a hospital unit and a neurological assessment was allegedly performed but no neurological deficits were noted despite continued complaints of pain and tingling.

The following day, Gardner was assessed by an orthopedic surgeon who found that she had no reflexes in her lower extremities, could barely move her feet and had no bowel or bladder control. Plaintiff was transferred to a spinal treatment center where she was given steroids and underwent emergency spinal fixation surgery. While Gardner regained some of her neurological function, she was left with loss of muscle in her buttocks and legs. She has also developed a "hammer toe" condition.

Plaintiff claimed that she was not properly assessed and treated for the injury she sustained with the result that she was left with neurological deficits which could have been avoided if they had been cared for and treated appropriately.

Conclusion:

Plaintiff's verdict for $1.9 million.

Case Name:	**Baker vs. Quinn**
Date:	7/16/98
Case Number:	A98A0325
Court:	State Court, Fulton County, Georgia

Case Synopsis:

Plaintiff went to a hospital for hernia surgery which resulted in paralysis from the waist down. Plaintiff and his wife filed suit against the surgeon and the anesthetist. Both parties entered into a verbal agreement whereby the Defendant's liability was limited to an amount between $600,000.00 and $1,600,000.00. After the jury entered a judgment of $5,650,000.00 the Plaintiffs and Defendants asserted different recollections of the verbal agreement.

Conclusion:

Verdict for the Plaintiffs in the amount of $5,650,000.00. The judge upheld the jury's verdict since there was apparently no agreement between the parties on the verbal liability limit.

Case Name: **Keats vs. Dr. Vijay Amano**
Date: 8/10/00
Case Number: 24C-99-002806
Court: Circuit Court, Baltimore City, Maryland

Case Synopsis:

Plaintiff sustained a perforated duodenum during balloon dilatation in an attempt to enter the small bowel. Plaintiff claimed that the balloon was improperly positioned with the result that the duodenum was perforated. The patient underwent several surgical procedures to repair the perforation and address complications. He died four months later of cardiac arrest. He was 76 years old at the time of his death.

Defendants denied fault and asserted that perforation is a known complication of the procedure and that the decision to repair the perforation was made in a timely fashion.

Conclusion: Plaintiff's verdict in the amount of $14.15 million.

Comments: Maryland's tort reform statutes apparently limit the amount of Plaintiff's damage to $300,000 in non-economic damages but otherwise cap the maximum judgment at $1,345,000.00.

Case Name:	**Tom and Vanna Colbert vs. Dr. Ken A. Smyth**
Date:	11/7/03
Case Number:	Unknown
Court:	Circuit Court, Anne Arundel County, Maryland

Case Synopsis:

Medical malpractice claim by the parents of a brain damaged boy who claimed that Dr. Ken A. Smyth acted below the standard of care and was negligent in his care and treatment of their now 10-year-old son. They filed suit in 2001 after a nurse who participated in the birth of the boy approached them at a family picnic and told them of acts, errors and omissions that she believed caused their son's brain damage. Patrick Colbert has an IQ of 49, suffers from severe learning disabilities and has no ability to care for himself.

Vanna Colbert went to her obstetrician for a routine prenatal checkup on November 9, 1992, during which it was determined that Patrick's heart was beating at more than 200 beats per minute, a life-threatening condition known as fetal tachycardia. She was rushed to Anne Arundel Medical Center, where an emergency Caesarean section at 12:24 p.m. When he was delivered, Patrick's heart was still beating at a very high rate and he was blue. Dr. Smyth gave Patrick oxygen by mask and tried to revive him by placing ice on his cheeks, but did not insert an oxygen tube down his breathing passage until 1:20 p.m., some 56 minutes after his birth. At 1:38 p.m. Dr. Smyth, at the suggestion of a nurse, administered a dose of a heart drug called adenosine. Within five minutes, Patrick's heart rate returned to normal and his color to a healthy pink. The Plaintiffs argued that oxygen deprivation for 80 minutes after the delivery led to severe and permanent brain damage.

The doctor and the Annapolis hospital denied any fault on their part and argued that other factors may have caused the boy's retardation.

Conclusion:

Plaintiffs' verdict for $6.4 million. The jury awarded $1.4 million for Patrick's future medical expenses, $3.5 million for his lost earning capacity, and $1.5 million for pain and suffering.

Case Name: **Fosley vs. OCC Diagnostic Systems, Inc.**

Date: 4/16/99
Case Number: 164506
Court: Circuit Court, Montgomery County, Maryland

Case Synopsis:

OCC Diagnostic Systems, Inc. reported Pap smear tests performed on Foster in April and December of 1992, as normal. The Plaintiff, age 36, was later diagnosed has having cervical cancer and underwent a radical hysterectomy. She also developed squamous cell carcinoma of the vagina and surrounding tissue.

Fosley and her husband sued the laboratory for negligently misreading the Pap smear slides which Plaintiffs claimed showed grossly abnormal cells. Plaintiff claimed that had the Pap smears been properly read and an appropriate referral made for treatment, a cone biopsy could have been performed and the development of the cancer stopped.

Fosley was 36-years-old at the time she was diagnosed and was working as a salesperson making approximately $25,000 annually. She now earns $19,000 with a new employer also doing sales work.

Conclusion:

Plaintiffs' verdict for $1.02 million, including $250,000 on the loss of consortium claim.

Case Name: **Lesa Waynell vs. Dr. G. Rucker, Trim Clinic and Louisiana Medical Mutual Insurance Company**

Date: 9/25/02

Case Number: 430149

Court: District Court, East Baton Rouge, Louisiana

Case Synopsis:

Medical malpractice claim was filed by the Plaintiff who suffered a stroke after being given Didrex pills at the Trim Clinic weight loss center by Dr. G. Rucker. Plaintiff claimed that the prescription was both stronger and in a greater dosage than allowed by the Louisiana Board of Medical Examiners.

Defendant denied that any act, error, or omission on their part caused or contributed to the Plaintiff's injuries.

Conclusion:

Plaintiff's verdict for $4.592 million reduced to $500,000 by state medical malpractice cap.

Case Name:	**Graham Breen vs. Baptist East Hospital**
	East and Dr. Marcia Coal
Date:	4/19/04
Case Number:	Unknown
Court:	Jefferson County, Kentucky

Case Synopsis:

Graham Breen and his family claimed that Dr. Marcia Coal and the nurses and staff at Baptist East Hospital negligently failed to exercise due care during the labor and delivery process with the result that he sustained permanent brain damage and needs constant care. The Plaintiffs further claimed that the brain damage that he sustained were the result of avoidable complications caused by medical malpractice during the delivery. Graham's injuries will necessitate 24-hour-a-day care for the rest of his life. He is now 5 years old.

Labor was induced on August 28th. Judy Breen testified that she was given multiple doses of Pitocin (brand name for the generic drug Oxytocin).

The Defendants denied that they were negligent and that the delivery took an unexpected turn at the last minute.

Conclusion:

Plaintiffs' verdict for $27.5 million.

Case Name:	**Lestor Layne, as Conservator**
	of Ron Frost, and Pamela Mixon,
	as Mother of Ron Frost vs. Baptist East Hospital
Date:	12/2/02
Case Number:	0-CI-01471
Court:	Division Six, Circuit Court, Jefferson County, Kentucky

Case Synopsis:

Medical Malpractice Claim - Brain Damage - Permanent Vegetative State - Pamela Mixon took her son Ron Frost, age 14, to Baptist East Hospital in Louisville, Kentucky for treatment of his broken left forearm sustained while playing football. Plaintiffs claimed that Ron's airway became obstructed during surgery the next morning. Dr. Eileen Jones was the anesthesiologist assigned to Ron's case. As a result of the alleged negligence of Dr. Jones, Ron sustained permanent brain damage and now exists in a near vegetative state. Plaintiffs claimed that the care provided to Ron at Baptist East was below the standard of care and that as a direct result, Ron was harmed.

Plaintiffs sought past and future medical expenses, lost earnings and future mental and physical suffering damages. The Defendants denied that any negligent act, error, or omission on their respective parts caused any harm to Ron.

Conclusion:

Baptist East Hospital settled before trial for an undisclosed sum and a jury awarded the Plaintiffs $12.1 million in damages.

Case Name: **Will Roberts vs. T.J. Samson Community Hospital, Dr. G. Newton and Dr. M. Bonner**

Date: 2/4/00

Case Number: 98cv44

Court: United States District Court for the Western District of Kentucky

Case Synopsis:

Medical malpractice - Plaintiff claimed that his penis and his left testicle were removed, without his consent, during surgery for an infection. Mr. Roberts was admitted to T.J. Samson Community Hospital on three occasions in 1997 for treatment of an infected cyst on one of his legs. The infection later spread to his groin, and he underwent surgery to remove the cyst and other infected tissue. Roberts claimed that he was never told that his penis and testicle might be removed and would not have consented to the surgery had he been informed of what Defendants intended to do to him.

Defendants claimed that the amputation was medically necessary and denied wrongdoing.

Conclusion:

Plaintiff's verdict awarding Will Roberts $1.9 million for pain and suffering and $449,832 for past and future medical bills. Mrs. Roberts was awarded $250,000 for loss of consortium.

Case Name: **Ralph Carter vs. Dr. Barbara Ramoski**
Date: 12/11/02
Case Number: 00-CV-1450G
Court: Superior Court, Suffolk County, Massachusetts

Case Synopsis:

Medical malpractice claim by Ralph Carter who claimed that Dr. Barbara Ramoski at Boston's Carney Hospital negligently performed a procedure on him to drain his bladder and as a direct result his bowel was perforated. The puncture was not immediately diagnosed, and he developed necrotizing fasciitis necessitating many surgeries to removed most of his stomach and abdominal muscles. The 74-year-old Mr. Kent was in the hospital for three months and ended up with a colostomy.

Conclusion:

Plaintiff's verdict for $7.1 million.

Case Name:	**Sara and Leonard Brown vs. Huntsville Hospital and Dr. John Mace**
Date:	5/13/04
Case Number:	CV-99-1417
Court:	Circuit Court, Madison County, Alabama

Case Synopsis:

On October 6, 1997, Sara Brown took her eleven-month-old son, Charlie, to the emergency room at Huntsville Hospital because he had a high fever, a high pulse rate, and trouble breathing. Dr. Mace, who was board-certified in family practice, was working in the emergency room when the Browns arrived at the hospital. Dr. Mace treated Charlie for croup, observed him for three hours, gave Sara a prescription for Charlie, and then released him to go home. After Sara left the hospital, she went to a Winn Dixie pharmacy to get Charlie's prescription filled. While at the pharmacy, Charlie went into respiratory arrest and then cardiac arrest. Emergency medical technicians, responding to a 911 emergency call, transported Charlie to Huntsville Hospital, where he was pronounced dead. An autopsy of Charlie indicated that he died of necrotizing tracheobronchitis (severe tracheitis and bronchitis), a severe infection of the trachea and bronchi that obstructed his airway.

The Plaintiffs sued Huntsville Hospital and Dr. Mace for medical malpractice. To prove medical negligence, the Plaintiffs offered expert medical testimony by Dr. Matt Webber, who was board-certified in pediatrics, in emergency medicine, and in pediatric emergency medicine, and Dr. Luke Kreplick, who was board-certified in emergency medicine. The Defendants objected to expert testimony from Dr. Webber and Dr. Kreplick on the ground that they were not "similarly situated" with Dr. Mace in that neither Dr. Webber nor Dr. Kreplick was board-certified in family practice as Dr. Mace was.

Conclusion:

Plaintiffs' verdict for $2 million.

Case Name:	**Weslyn vs. Cleveland Clinic Foundation**
Date:	8/31/97
Case Number:	301267
Court:	Court of Common Pleas of Cuyahoga County

Case Synopsis:

Mrs. Weslyn, age 58, underwent an elective surgery for a deviated septum at the recommendation of her otolaryngologist, who said that he would perform the surgery but did not. The anesthesiologist left the operating room after the surgery was begun and left Mrs. Weslyn under the care of a CRNA who removed her from the ventilator prematurely. Mrs. Wesley went into cardiac arrest and suffered brain damage which left her in a persistent vegetative requiring 24-hour-care. Plaintiff claimed that Weslyn was negligently removed from the ventilator and asserted fraud and battery claims.

Conclusion:

Verdict for Plaintiff for $14.5 million, including $11 million in compensatory damages and $3.5 million in punitive damages.

Case Name: **Jana, Greg, and Kaylen Rinds vs. Dr. Stiles Cullen**
Date: 2/6/04
Case Number: Unknown
Court: Circuit Court, Davies County, Indiana

Case Synopsis:

Medical malpractice claim by the parents of Kaylen Rinds who claimed that Dr. Stiles Cullen acted below the standard of care when he failed to call for assistance when he was notified that Kaylen's heart rate had fallen from 150 to 90 beats a minute. Instead, they proceeded to the hospital before calling for assistance from Dr. Vaun Forsythe to perform a C-section on Jana who had suffered a placenta abrupta at approximately 3:30 a.m. on February 15, 2000. The Plaintiffs claimed that Kaylen suffered severe brain damage and is in a persistent vegetative state and is taken care of 24 hours and day 7 days a week by Greg Rinds. The Plaintiffs claimed that he kept saying: "Why didn't I call the surgery team in when I called you on the phone."

Cullen denied that he acted below the standard of care or made any admissions of fault after the delivery.

Conclusion:

Plaintiffs' verdict for $7 million - $3.2 million to Jana Rinds, $2.3 million to Kaylen Rinds and $1.5 million to Greg Rinds – The verdict outcome was limited to $1.25 million by InBelinda's cap of $1.25 million in medical malpractice cases.

Case Name:	**Peters vs. Providence St. Vincent Medical Center**
Date:	2/5/99
Case Number:	9701-00543
Court:	District Court, Multnomah County, Oregon

Case Synopsis:

Denise Peters was examined for abdominal pain in 1996. During exploratory surgery, the anesthesiologist inserted a catheter into the wall of her heart when he attempted to insert a central venous catheter into her neck. The pericardial sac around her heart filed with fluid and her heart stopped beating. Mrs. Peters sustained severe brain damage and now requires 24-hour care. The Plaintiffs claimed that hospital personnel failed to follow procedures by not monitoring the placement of the catheter before inserting fluids and that the doctors had failed to detect and respond to the improper insertion of the catheter and the buildup of fluids around Peters' heart.

Conclusion:

Plaintiffs' verdict for $15.77 million for Mrs. Peters and $2 million for Mr. Peters against St. Vincent only.

Case Name: **Lana Knowles vs. Lawrence Belling,**
MD, Victor Warner,
MD, and Queen City Vascular and General Surgeons

Date: 3/15/04

Case Number: A-01-02321

Court: Court of Common Pleas, Hamilton County, Ohio

Case Synopsis:

Medical Malpractice - Surgery - Necrotizing Fasciitis

Plaintiff entered Mercy Franciscan Mt. Airy Hospital in Cincinnati, Ohio on February 14, 2001, with complaints of severe right lower quadrant abdominal pain. Defendant, Belling, removed Plaintiff's appendix on February 15, 2001.

Belling was off for the weekend and Defendant Warner, another surgeon in Defendant Queen City General and Vascular Surgeons was responsible for Plaintiff's care. Despite two CT-scans showing the presence of necrotizing fasciitis and a radiology report confirming this diagnosis, Warner did not perform surgery or modify antibiotic treatment.

On Monday February 19, 2001, Belling took Plaintiff to surgery and removed tissue but not the infected fascia. Plaintiff expired after a third debridement surgery on February 21, 2001.

Conclusion:

Plaintiff's verdict for $4,108,132.14. Plaintiff had requested that the jury award $3,000,000.

Case Name:	**Stanton vs. New York City**
	Health and Hospitals Corporation
Date:	12/7/98
Case Number:	Unknown
Court:	Supreme Court, Queens County, New York

Case Synopsis:

Plaintiffs claimed that Defendants mishandled the breach birth of their daughter, Tina, who was born at Defendant's hospital in November 1998. Plaintiffs claimed that the child should have been delivered by Caesarian section rather that vaginally. Despite signs of fetal distress, Defendant allowed the child to be delivered vaginally with the result that there was cord compression and the baby's head became trapped in the mother's uterus. An attempt at a forceps delivery was unsuccessful and drugs were given to relax the uterus, but it took ten minutes to deliver the baby with the result that it sustained severe asphyxiation with resulting brain damage. Defendants denied any negligence.

Conclusion:

Verdict for Plaintiffs for $116 million reduced to a present value of approximately $25 million.

Case Name: **Karen vs. Palladow**
Date: 2/6/98
Case Number: 93-914
Court: Circuit Court, Macomb County, Michigan

Case Synopsis:

Karen, age 44, noticed nipple retraction and a possible lump in her right breast. In March 1991, she had a mammogram performed and it was interpreted as being normal. Four months later another mammogram was performed after she decided that the lump had increased in size. Again, the radiologist interpreted the mammogram as normal. In December 1991, a third mammogram was performed. This time the same radiologist interpreted the mammogram as suspicious. A biopsy was performed, and the tissues diagnosed as being malignant. It was determined that the cancer had spread to Karen's lymph nodes. By 1997 the cancer had spread to Karen's hip, and she was given only two years to live. Karen and her husband brought suit against the radiologist claiming negligence on his part in failing to properly interpret the mammograms. Plaintiffs claimed that Karen would have had more than a 90% chance of survival had her cancer been diagnosed and treated in March 1991.

Conclusion:

Verdict for Plaintiff for $1.75 million.

Case Name: **Myra Davis vs. United Health Services Hospital, Inc.**
Date: 5/14/98
Case Number: 95-0177
Court: Supreme Court, Broome County, New York

Case Synopsis:

Myra Davis began experiencing visual disturbances and headaches when she was seven months pregnant for which she was hospitalized. On the second day of the hospitalization, she suffered a grand mal seizure. She was found in an unresponsive state, and after time, her obstetrician and her neurologist were contacted. Dilantin was ordered but not given. Plaintiff then suffered two more seizures. An emergency C-section was performed, and her baby was born with depressed Apgar scores. He later developed an E. coli infection in the hospital nursery and went into septic shock. The child then developed spastic quadriplegia. He cannot sit, stand, or speak and is institutionalized. Plaintiff alleged that the baby suffered fetal hypoxia during the seizures that set the stage for the infectious process. The life expectancy of the child was contested by the parties.

Conclusion:

Verdict for Plaintiffs for $103.13 million.

Case Name:	James Tatum, as Administrator of Estate of Donna Tatum (deceased) vs. J. William James, M.D. and Greg Moroney, Certified Registered Nurse Anesthetist
Date:	7/9/99
Case Number:	78,905
Court:	Ellis District Court, Kansas

Case Synopsis:

Medical Malpractice - Wrongful Death - Anesthesia - Administrator of estate of his wife and mother of his surviving minor child filed medical malpractice suit against the obstetrician and certified registered nurse who delivered deceased's baby. The deceased died as a result of a reaction to anesthesia during a routine cesarean section on September 11, 1994, at Hays Medical Center. For the delivery, the deceased's regular doctor was unavailable, so Defendant assisted, as the patient's labor did not progress in a normal manner. The Defendant ordered the anesthesia services of a certified nurse anesthetist Greg Maroney. The nurse went over the patient's options with her before performing the procedure, as required. The patient chose to have a spinal instead of General anesthetic. The facts of the actual surgery are in dispute, as the Plaintiff's version of events was different from the Defendant's. The Plaintiff stated that Dr. James made an incision about 4-6 inches deep and the patient complained that she could feel the pain. The Plaintiff further stated that a mask was then placed over her face and he was removed from the operating room. Dr. James stated that he only nicked the patient's skin on the first incision and immediately discontinued the surgery, because the spinal revealed spots of blood. He further testified that the nurse then selected a general anesthesia and placed an oxygen mask on the patient, which helps a patient's safety during surgery. The doctor then stated that the nurse gave the patient a muscle relaxant, Sodium Penathol, a sleeping agent and Anectine, which paralyzes the muscles. The nurse, with the help of another nurse, attempted to intubate the patient to help her breathe. When the doctor made the last cut to remove the infant, that he found red blood in the placenta, which is an indication that the patient is not receiving enough oxygen. The doctor testified that he had no idea that the patient had not been correctly intubated until this time. The tube was then pulled, and the patient was masked, and the patient was bagged in an effort to keep her breathing until the baby was delivered and also following the procedure. The patient was then given more Ancetine and another effort to intubate was made. All efforts made by hospital personnel to resuscitate the patient were unsuccessful, and she died of hypoxia.

Conclusion:

The Plaintiff was awarded $2,007,385.77 in total damages.

Case Name: **Harvey Rast vs. Mercy Memorial Health Center**
Date: 3/3/00
Case Number: 99-CV-245
Court: United States District Court for the Eastern District of Oklahoma

Case Synopsis:

On July 5, 1997, at 4:00 a.m., Harvey Rast, a 47-year-old manager and part owner of the Sirloin Stockade went to the hospital due to suffering from severe abdominal pain. While being treated in the emergency room he was given painkillers and tranquilizers. By 6:00 a.m. a nurse in the emergency room noted that the Plaintiff was shaking uncontrollably, yet at 6:10 he was released from the hospital and given a diagnosis of the flu.

The Plaintiff later returned to the hospital and underwent emergency surgery to remove his small intestine and half of his large bowel due to a blood clot, which had lodged in the artery supplying blood to his intestines.

Defendant denied wrongdoing and claimed the medical care given met the highest standards of care. Defendant also alleged that all test results and examination of Mr. Rast were normal.

Conclusion:

Jury returned with verdict at 6:10 p.m. VERDICT: Finding in favor of Plaintiff Harvey Rast in the amount of $5,000,000.00 and Plaintiff Viola Rast in the amount of $1,000,000.00 and against Brent Gillis, D.O. and Emergency Physicians of Southern Oklahoma. The EMTALA claim against Mercy Memorial Health Center was dismissed at trial.

Case Name:	**Najee Imes vs. New York City**
	Health and Hospitals Corporation
Date:	3/31/98
Case Number:	670 N.Y.S.2d 486 (A.D. 1 Dept. 1998)
Court:	Supreme Court, Appellate Division, First Department

Case Synopsis:

Sonya Imes, the Plaintiff-mother complained to her obstetrician, Defendant Reyes Vendez, M.D., at a scheduled office visit, that she was having labor pains although she was two months short of carrying to full term. She was sent home but told to go to the hospital if the pains continued. Later that evening she did go to the hospital because her contractions were stronger, and she was bleeding. She went to one hospital and was then sent to another. After waiting over six hours, the Defendant determined Plaintiff was indeed going into delivery and a Caesarean section was performed. The child weighed only 3 pounds and suffers from cerebral palsy due to hypoxia. Union Hospital was negligent in failing to refer Ms. Imes to the emergency room or an obstetrical area when it had knowledge that Dr. Vendez was unavailable.

Conclusion:

Plaintiff's verdict for $4,796,483 for future custodial care and $3,157,469 for loss of future earnings.

Case Name: **Edna Viren vs. Cleveland Clinic Foundation**
Date: 11/23/98
Case Number: 72838
Court: Court of Common Pleas, Cuyahoga County, Ohio

Case Synopsis:

In April of 1995, the Plaintiff, who was sixty years old, went to Defendant with a sinus infection. She was referred to a specialist in Ear, Nose and Throat Department at the clinic, who noted that there was no infection. The specialist diagnosed that the Plaintiff had a deviated septum in her nose and stated that she would need surgery. The doctor advised the Plaintiff that he would have the help of medical residents during the surgery and also told of the risks and benefits of the operation, and the Plaintiff did not object. The Plaintiff, however, did not sign a medical consent form for the surgery. On the day of the surgery, the specialist was also to perform four other surgeries and the anesthesiologist moved from room to room to assist. Also present in the operating room was a nurse anesthetist and the Chief Resident of the ENT Department. The specialist was noted as the doctor of record for the procedure, but the Chief resident filled in for him during the procedure, while the specialist went to other rooms. The Plaintiff was intubated during the surgery to ensure proper breathing and the surgery was uneventful; the specialist could not recall if he was present when the Plaintiff was extubated. After the surgery, the Plaintiff's heart rate dropped, and she was reintubated shortly after she was resuscitated. She remains in a vegetative state.

Conclusion:

Plaintiff's verdict for $9,600,000 in compensatory damages, $1,300,000 to the husband for loss of consortium and $3,500,000 in punitive damages.

Case Name:	**Edina A. Manson vs. Hickston**
Date:	5/7/99
Case Number:	9465/96
Court:	Supreme Court, Kings County, New York

Case Synopsis:

Plaintiff complains of failure to properly address hypovolemia after uterine fibroid surgery with resulting permanent brain damage and blindness. Plaintiff, Edina A. Manson, age 35, was admitted to Lutheran Medical Center in New York on December 9, 1994, to undergo abdominal surgery to remove uterine fibroids by Dr. Hickston. After the surgery, an IV solution containing dextrose was administered to replace fluids lost during the surgery. The fact that Ms. Manson had become hypovolemic was not detected in time to prevent permanent brain damage and impairment of her vision to the point that she is nearly blind. Before the surgery, Ms. Manson was an administrative assistant for the New York City Housing Authority. She is now unable to work. Plaintiff claimed that she should have been given a saline and electrolyte-based intravenous solution.

Conclusion:

Dr. Hickston settled the claim against him for $1.8 million during trial and the jury returned a verdict in Ms. Manson' favor in the amount of $19.08 million and awarded her husband $450,000 with a finding that the hospital was 40% responsible for the injuries and damages sustained.

Case Name: **Abbey Miller, et al. vs. New York City**
Health and Hospital Corp.
Date: 6/30/99
Case Number: 14089/86
Court: Supreme Court, Bronx County, New York

Case Synopsis:

Medical malpractice – Abbey Miller presented to Jacobi Medical Center in the Bronx for delivery of her third child suffering from pre-eclampsia. Despite the fact that both of her first children were delivered by Cesarean section because of the same condition, she was allowed to progress toward a vaginal delivery. Eventually a C-section was performed but the Plaintiff's baby, Joel Miller, had already sustained permanent brain damage and was left with mild cerebral palsy that does not affect his intelligence but left him with a limp and diminished use of one hand.

Conclusion:

Plaintiffs' verdict for $7.44 million.

Case Name:	**Feather vs. Sheagal**
Date:	6/30/00
Case Number:	4129/93
Court:	Supreme Court, King County, New York

Case Synopsis:

Plaintiff complains of failure to diagnose and treat congenital aneurysm in 23-year-old elevator mechanic who presented at Long Island College Hospital in 1991, complaining of severe pain in his back and a headache. Plaintiffs claimed that Defendants failed to conduct a proper differential diagnosis and did not conduct a proper neurological examination of Mr. Feather. He died several hours after being admitted to the hospital from a ruptured cerebral aneurysm.

Conclusion:

Plaintiffs' verdict for $41.44 million.

Case Name: **Andrew Balleras vs. City of New York**
Health and Hospitals Corp.
Date: 5/17/01
Case Number: Unknown
Court: Supreme Court, New York County, New York

Case Synopsis:

Brain damage was sustained by a newborn that contracted bacterial meningitis from his mother at birth. A test for the bacteria was ordered a day late, resulting in a corresponding delay in treatment of the child. There was also a daylong delay in returning the test results from a lab, and another 24 hours elapsed before Andrew was given antibiotics to combat the group B-strep he contracted from his mother.

Conclusion:

Plaintiffs for $107.8 million

Case Name: **Frederick Smith vs. Bronx Lebanon Hospital**
Date: 1/24/03
Case Number: 14032/1994
Court: Supreme Court, New York County, New York

Case Synopsis:

19-year-old Frederick Smith was taken to Bronx Lebanon Hospital on September 23, 1991, suffering from pneumonia symptoms. Hospital personnel were aware that the boy suffered from sickle-cell anemia and concentrated on that diagnosis rather than the possibility that the boy's chest pain was related to his sickle-cell anemia. Because the boy's blood could not provide adequate oxygen to his brain, he sustained brain damage which left him a profoundly retarded spastic quadriplegic. He is bedridden and his communication is basically limited to blinking his eyes.

Conclusion:

Plaintiff's verdict for $20.9 million.

Case Name: **Donald and Brandi Sexton vs. John Doe(s)**
and Fletcher Allen Health Care Center
Date: 8/31/98
Case Number: SO479-96-CnC
Court: Superior Court of Chittenden County

Case Synopsis:

Defendant is charged with failure to properly monitor post-operative recovery period after spinal surgery to remove a tumor. Plaintiff complained of numbness in his feet. No action was taken for a two day period. Eventually an MRI was performed which revealed a buildup of fluid that was putting pressure on his spinal cord. Emergency surgery to relieve the pressure was unsuccessful with the result that Plaintiff was left with permanent paralysis.

Conclusion:

Verdict for Donovan Sexton for $1,579,375 and for Mrs. Sexton for $500,000 for loss of consortium.

Case Name: **Dondi Wade vs. Phillip Shapiro, D.O.**
Date: 10/21/99
Case Number: Unknown
Court: Circuit Court, Wayne County, Michigan

Case Synopsis:

Medical malpractice - Plaintiff claimed that Defendant performed a wrong level back surgery (L3-L4 instead of an L4-L5) and then concealed his error for nearly two years. As a result, Plaintiff became totally disabled and eventually underwent the proper surgery.

Ms. Wade, a 40-year-old single waitress with the Marriott Corporation for 16 years, developed a herniated disc at L4-L5 in 1993. Although surgery was indicated, Dr. Shapiro did the surgery at the wrong level (L3-L4 instead of L4-L5). Then, even though radiographic testing demonstrated the surgery was done at the wrong level, Shapiro put Wade on conservative therapy for over two years, causing additional extensive damage. Shapiro did not inform Plaintiff of his mistake and explained away the concerns she voiced to him after she learned of inconsistencies from her physical therapist nearly two years later. The proper course would have been for Shapiro to immediately inform the patient and reschedule the patient for surgery upon learning of the initial error.

Conclusion:

Plaintiff's verdict for $4 million.

Case Name: **DeAngelo vs. Thomas Jefferson University Hospital**
Date: 12/19/98
Case Number: Unknown
Court: Court of Common Pleas, Philadelphia County, Pennsylvania

Case Synopsis:

Plaintiff's decedent was diagnosed as having an atrial myxoma penetrating the left ventricle and left atrial chambers of the heart. During exploratory surgery, the surgeon attempted to resect and remove the mass with the result that particles of the mass were released causing many small stokes which left the patient in a semi-vegetative state for nearly two years before her death. Plaintiff claimed that the patient should never have been operated on to remove the mass because it was inoperable and that preoperative tests revealed that surgery was futile. Plaintiff also claimed that Defendants did not inform the patient that she had other options.

Conclusion:

Verdict for Plaintiffs for $5.9 million.

Case Name:	**Welston vs. Greg Mc Phearson and Spectrascan Imaging Services Inc.**
Date:	12/13/98
Case Number:	96-C-1462JV
Court:	Court of Common Pleas, Lehigh County, Pennsylvania

Case Synopsis:

Plaintiff went to her gynecologist for a routine checkup. During the examination Dr. Mc Phearson found a lump in her breast and sent her to Spectrascan Imaging Services Inc. for a mammogram which was reported to show no abnormalities. Eight months later she went back to Dr. Mc Phearson because the lump had enlarged to the point that she could feel it. She was referred to a surgeon who determined that the lump was cancer and that it had spread into her lymph nodes. Despite chemotherapy, Ms. Welston is not expected to live. Ms. Welston sued Dr. Mc Phearson and Spectrascan, charging that Spectrascan was negligent because its technologist sent Ms. Welston's mammogram to the wrong file in Dr. Mc Phearson's office. The mammogram, because it had been ordered after the discovery of a lump, should have been routed directly to Dr. Mc Phearson. When it was sent to the normal pile of mammogram reports, no surgical consultation was ordered, and thus the nature of the lump was not discovered. At trial, Dr. Mc Phearson admitted problems with his office procedures. Spectrascan denied any negligence.

Conclusion:

Verdict for Plaintiff for $33.1 million.

Case Name: **Ethyl Thurgood vs. Dr. Robert Quinton**
Date: 9/24/99
Case Number: 98-CV-860
Court: United States District Court for the Middle District of Pennsylvania

Case Synopsis:

Negligence in the performance of an operation to remove the lower lobe of Plaintiff's left lung. Plaintiff underwent the surgery in August 1996, when she was 50 years old. Plaintiff alleged that Quinton cut a hole in her diaphragm that he allegedly repaired. Plaintiff's stomach later ruptured through the cut in the diaphragm, spilling the contents of the stomach into the lung, which had to be removed.

Conclusion:

Plaintiff's verdict for $16.8 million, assessing 55% of the liability to Dr. Quinton and 45% to the other Defendants.

Case Name:	**Mark Alston (guardian for Alyssa Vladmir)**
	vs. Dr. Nick D'Anna
Date:	12/4/00
Case Number:	Sept. Term 1997, No. 3379
Court:	Court of Common Pleas, Philadelphia County, Pennsylvania

Case Synopsis:

Plaintiff claimed that Dr. Nick D'Anna damaged Alyssa Vladmir's phrenic nerve during an unsuccessful operation on September 26, 1995, to close the ductus arteriosis at St. Seth's Hospital in Bethlehem, Pennsylvania. As a result, Alyssa is now profoundly retarded, wheelchair bound, cannot eat and cannot speak. The child was then transferred to St. Christopher's Hospital in Philadelphia where a second operation successfully closed the ductus arteriosis but where a nurse mistakenly inserted an arterial line into the wrong artery of her left arm with the result that blood flow was stopped to the arm and it had to be amputated.

Plaintiff claimed that Dr. D'Anna was not well enough trained or experienced to perform the operation and that as a direct result, Alyssa was seriously harmed by the operation he attempted to perform on her.

Defendants claimed that Alyssa's retardation and other problems were caused by the fact that she was born at 26 weeks gestation and not by any act, error or omission on the part of Dr. D'Anna.

Conclusion:

Plaintiff's verdict for $100 million including $90 million in damages as a result of the alleged negligence of St. Seth's and Dr. D'Anna.

Case Name: **Webster vs. Collins**
Date: 5/10/01
Case Number: 3833
Court: Court of Common Pleas, Philadelphia County, Pennsylvania

Case Synopsis:

Plaintiff's decedent died from the loss of blood after an egg-retrieval procedure performed in preparation for an in vitro fertilization procedure. The woman presented at another doctor's office later in the day complaining of blood loss but was not seen for 90 minutes despite the fact that he was told that she was bleeding and that her blood pressure was dropping and that she was disoriented. She was later admitted to a hospital where it was determined that she had lost three-fourths of her blood volume and where attempts to stem her loss of blood were unsuccessful.

Conclusion:

Plaintiff verdict for $25 million with a finding that the physician who performed the egg-retrieval procedure was 25% at fault for her death.

Case Name:	**Estate of Robert Mason vs. St. Mary Medical Center, Langhorne Physician Services and Dr. Gary Carrasco**
Date:	12/5/02
Case Number:	Unknown
Court:	Court of Common Pleas, Bucks County, Pennsylvania

Case Synopsis:

Medical malpractice claims relating to the failure by Dr. Gary Carrasco to properly diagnose and treat the heart attack that Bucks County business executive Robert Mason, 39, was having when he presented at the St. Mary Medical Center on Sept. 28, 1994. Mason was found dead in his car by a jogger several hours later near his home. After blood tests and an electrocardiogram, he spent ten minutes with an emergency room doctor, court records say.

Robert Mason was earning more than $2 million per year as president of a Bristol dental and orthodontic supply firm. His family claimed that, had he lived, Mason might have earned an additional $66 million over his lifetime according to one of his family's expert witnesses.

It is not known at this time what defenses were asserted by the defense, but it was probably a combination of denial of negligence on the part of the Defendants plus a claim that there was no causal connection between any act, error or omission on the part of Dr. Carrasco.

Conclusion:

Settled for $15 million.

Comments:

One of the problems with proposed tort reform legislation is that it would cap the damages that can be awarded to a Plaintiff in a medical malpractice case, essentially depriving someone like Mr. Mason's family of adequate compensation for the loss sustained as a result of the substandard care provided to him at the hospital.

CHAPTER 20

Larren Legal Case Assessment

On Tuesday, August 14th, five months after Amy's botched surgery, we received a copy of the petition from our attorneys. During unscheduled but frequent talks with them, we discussed the preliminary evaluation of our case against responsible parties. There is the side of the case that our attorneys are constructing through the discovery phase, but I am limited on what I can cover on that due to the case is still open. The best way to summarize our case is by starting from the discharge summary portion of the medical records, as laid out – in its entirety – by Dr. Keel herself.

```
ADMITTING DIAGNOSES:
    1. Spontaneous miscarriage x2.
    2. Abnormal ultrasound suggestive of uterine septum.

DISCHARGE DIAGNOSES:
    1. Status post hysteroscopy, laparoscopy and repair of vena
       cava tear on 03/07/20xx.
    2. Status post exploratory thoracotomy and repair of
       subclavian artery perforation on 03/07/20xx.
```

3. Status post abdominal re-exploration with repair of mesenteric arterial bleeding, repair of transverse colon perforation, repair of left proximal iliac artery with graft on 03/08/20xx.

HOSPITAL COURSE:
This is a 23-year-old, white female **who has had 2 miscarriages**. She has had an ultrasound that showed what appeared to be either a bicornuate uterus or a uterine septum. To evaluate this intrauterine abnormality, she underwent a hysterosalpingogram. At the time of the hysterosalpingogram, there was residual placental and fetal tissue which made the hysterosalpingogram un-interpretable. There was a filling defect in the uterus, but it made it difficult to evaluate the cavity for septum or bicornuate uterus. The patient was counselled as to alternatives at this point and as the HSG was very uncomfortable for her, she did not want to go through with that procedure again. If there were a septum, she would need that ablated in order to improve her obstetric outcomes. She was admitted on 03/07/20xx for hysteroscopy with possible ablation of intrauterine septum, along with laparoscopy. The hysteroscopy was uneventful, and an intrauterine septum was seen. The septum did appear somewhat thick and to confirm that it was indeed a septum and also to make lasering of the septum safe, a laparoscopy was performed. As in the operative report, at the time of laparoscopy, there was blood in the pelvis and in the abdomen which was concerning for hemorrhage. The patient was hemodynamically stable, but as the reason for the blood was not immediately evident at laparoscopy, I felt that proceeding immediately to laparotomy was indicated. This was performed quickly, and the belly was entered as dictated in the operative report. My partner, Dr. Finch, was called to assist with the procedure and arrived promptly. We identified a retroperitoneal bleeder, and this was quickly controlled until a cardiovascular surgeon could arrive. Dr. Milton was available and arrived to repair what seemed to be an intra-

vena caval puncture. During her surgery, she lost approximately 2000 cubic centimeters of blood. Dr. Lister, the anesthesiologist, appropriately had placed an extra-venous access in her arm, in addition to a central line. After completion of these procedures, she went to recovery. She arrived in recovery at approximately 12:10 p.m. Following her arrival in recovery and after I was assured that she was stable, I did discuss the procedure and the vena cava tear with the patient's **husband and family**. I then returned to the recovery room to reassess the patient and she continued to be stable. On review of her chest x-ray, after placement of the central line intraoperatively, there seemed to be some fluid in the pleural cavity on the side of the central line. The line had been used intraoperatively for blood only and was not being used in recovery at this point to my knowledge. I took the x-ray down to Dr. Hallund who reviewed it and said there was definitely fluid in this area and that it was not a pneumothorax. After discussing the situation with the line with Dr. Lister who had placed the line, he recommended that we discontinue it. **At about 13:45, the line was discontinued**, and pressure was applied. Immediately upon removing the catheter, the neck began to swell and firm pressure was continued to be held. Dr. Lister was paged at this point. Dr. Kane was at the bedside as he was immediately available. I arrived at this time also and it appeared that the patient had had a vascular injury from her central line. A right chest tube was placed by Dr. West and then the patient was taken immediately by Dr. Wales and Dr. West for thoracotomy and repair of subclavian artery perforation. While the patient was en route to the operating room, I returned to the waiting room to find the patient's family. The volunteers indicated that the husband had gone to eat lunch. I went to the lunchroom and the snack bar and could not find him. I returned to the operating room and had my nursing staff call the patient's emergency contact numbers to have the husband return. As I was returning back to the operating room, I did meet the patient's husband in the concourse on the way back up to the operating room. I explained to him Amy's situation at this point and what events had occurred at this time. He returned to the waiting room and I returned to the operating room. Following the thoracotomy, she was recovered as usual and then admitted to the intensive care unit. I had called Dr. Merle Edwards to assist with her care and he did evaluate the patient in recovery and followed her throughout her admission. On March 7th, Dr. Wales ordered a Swan-Ganz placed by cardiology because the patient was having hypotension. Dr. Ferris placed the Swan-Ganz at that time. On the morning of 03/08/20xx, the patient's abdomen became much more distended and tense. She continued to have a blood pressure systolic of 100. Dr. Milton and I evaluated her abdomen. Dr. Wales was also present, and we agreed that re-exploration was indicated as it appeared that she had continued intraabdominal bleeding. Dr. Milton re-explored her and repaired mesenteric artery bleeding. He also found through-and-through left iliac artery tear, which was repaired with a graft. **Apparently, what was initially thought to be an anterior vena cava tear was a through-and-through left iliac artery tear**. There was also a traverse colon perforation that was repaired at this time. Prior to this re-exploration, I had discussed the current problem with the patient's husband and her mother. On the evening of 03/08/20xx, the patient's condition improved, and she was no longer hypotensive. She was hemodynamically stable. On 03/09/20xx, she continued to improve. On 03/10/20xx, Dr. Milton discontinued her dopamine and at that point she also had developed some moderate vulvar edema, probably from just third spacing of fluid and after examining the edema, I recommended ice for the next 24 hours. This did improve on its own. She continued to do well and on March 11th, was placed on flow-by and eventually extubated. On March 12th, she continued to be stable, but her abdomen appeared to have an ileus, possibly due to morphine. Her pain medicines were changed and she was started on a liquid diet. Physical therapy was ordered to help the patient up in a chair and to eventually start ambulating. A dietary consult was also ordered to help with foods to prevent nausea and encourage oral intake. On March 13th, she was transferred to 8-West out of the ICU. On March 14th, her chest tube was pulled. She was continuing to tolerate oral feeding and on March 14th, had a small bowel movement. Her Foley was discontinued on March 14th. On the evening of March 14th, the patient had a large amount of emesis. Dr. Milton attempted to place a nasogastric tube, but the patient pulled it out. After a discussion that he indicates in the chart he had with the family, they agreed to leave the tube out, but make her (take) nothing by mouth until the abdominal exam improved. On March 15th, she had developed some pain in her left knee. Apparently, she told the nurses she had injured this knee sometime in the past, but it was somewhat swollen. An x-ray was obtained, which was normal. The knee was iced at this time. She continued to have nausea over the next 24 hours. It did gradually improve. On March 16th, the patient reported that her knee pain was better and pretty much had resolved. She had passed flatus and had good bowel sounds. She had an NG at this time that was clamped. She continued to have physical therapy to assist with ambulation. Over the next few days, she continued to have some abdominal distension. There was concern over her abdominal exam, but she was having bowel movements. She had an abdominal series on March 17th that showed an ileus, but no bowel obstruction. At that time, her NG was discontinued, and she was kept n.p.o. for the next few shifts. On March 18th, she was starting to take oral again and although her abdomen was somewhat distended, it seemed improved. On March 19th, she was tolerating p.o. well. Her antibiotics were discontinued, and her intravenous fluids were discontinued. She was encouraged to take oral nutrition. Over the next few days, we worked primarily on strength by encouraging her to ambulate. On March 22nd, her staples were partially discontinued. This was somewhat distressful for her and on my arrival that day, she was crying about the staple removal. The nurses had reported that the patient had seemed at times to be somewhat lethargic and poorly motivated to ambulate. I discussed this at length with her husband. He reports that he feels she will do better when she gets home to her usual environment. I did advise her that if she developed any signs of depression to notify us. On March 22nd, she was ready for discharge home. She was advised to follow up with Dr. Milton, Dr. Keel and Dr. Wales in 1 month. She was given a walker for home use, primarily because she still had some problems with the left knee buckling from an old injury. She was given instructions to call for temperature greater than 100, worsening pain control, or any other concerns.

The information provided by Dr. Keel is inclusive and provides a decent basis as to what occurred on March 7th, from a clinical standpoint, but is not entirely without error – at least from what I know some of the facts to be. Allow me to take a moment to draw out some of these errors from the above discharge summary. The bold text that I have included within the above Hospital Course transcript represents statements which I have determined to be inaccurate.

First, Dr. Keel contends that Amy suffered two spontaneous miscarriages, when in fact, only the first miscarriage was spontaneous. The second miscarriage was aided, if not caused by, the HSG that took place in December, three months prior to the botched surgery. An ER doctor from University Hospital, and even Dr. Keel herself in a conversation with me on the day of an emergency D&C performed at the same hospital, concluded that the HSG was likely to have caused the second miscarriage.

Second, Dr. Keel states that she discussed the vena cava tear with me and the family, but the family was not yet aware of any injury at this time and certainly was not at the hospital. This may be just a simple misstatement by the doctor, but the fact is she was only dealing with me at this time – not the family.

Third, Dr. Keel says that the central line was discontinued at 1:45p.m. This may be true, but what the doctor omits is the fact that discovery has determined that Dr. Lister was made aware of the chest cavity filling by the central line before 1:00 p.m. and ordered the discontinuing of the line accordingly by calling the same order down to the hospital staff in the recovery room with Amy. Dr. Keel overruled Dr. Lister without his knowing, and as a result Amy continued receiving the blood fluids for an additional 45 minutes before the central line was actually discontinued. This is one of the reasons our petition lists misconduct as a complaint against Dr. Keel.

Fourth, Dr. Keel minimizes the internal trauma by claiming that "what was initially thought to be an anterior vena cava tear was a through-and-through left iliac artery tear." Actually, there were both injuries present. After his second surgery on Amy on March 8th, Dr. Milton explained the procedure to the family and said that the initial injury was deeper than they had realized, holding his fingers about 6 inches apart. He said that during the earlier surgery he repaired the vena cava, or the blood vessel closer to the surface of her abdominal wall, but the one he had just repaired in this follow-up surgery was deeper than the first and was suspect to ongoing internal bleeding overnight. This indicates that there was damage to both the anterior and interior vena cava. Dr. Milton further admitted in this conversation that Amy's left iliac artery was damaged and was also bleeding internally, which he also repaired in the follow-up surgery. The left iliac artery feeds blood to the left leg, and damage to this artery was suspect as to why on the evening of March 7th, Amy's left foot was very cold even as her right foot was warm.

Fifth, Dr. Keel claims that on March 15th, Amy "developed" some pain in her left knee and told the nurses she had injured this knee sometime in the past. The truth is, Dr. Keel went away on vacation on March 9th and returned to the hospital on March 22nd, the day of Amy's discharge. Amy's leg pain didn't develop on the 15th. It was a problem for her when she first regained consciousness. Amy did not tell the nurses that she injured this knee before in the past. I, thinking aloud, could not figure out why it was swollen and commented about the strain injury that occurred on this knee very long ago when Amy was a CNA. Evidence suggested that the knee had a fresh and more recent contusive impact injury, and the fact that I was told that the x-rays were normal didn't make sense with the substantial swelling we were seeing at that time. It is very curious why the doctor says the knee was "somewhat" swollen, when truthfully it was "very, very" swollen. Also, we would learn that in fact, the knee x-rays were indeed not normal, as was substantiated by an ER visit to Lakeside North Hospital on Sunday, April 1st, and again by an orthopedic physician.

Sixth, Dr. Keel states that the knee problem was resolved on March 16th, and that Amy said it was better. The truth is entirely opposite of Dr. Keel's statement; not only did Amy deny the knee was better, but it also became increasingly worse. In fact, we were all suspicious and disturbed as to why no medical member seemed to be as concerned about it as Amy, me, or any of the family for that matter. To this day, Amy still has problems with her left knee.

Next, Dr. Keel says in this discharge summary that she discussed at length with me Amy's depressive state of mind. Dr. Keel had just returned from her vacation and was trying to get "caught up" on matters pertaining to Amy. We had not seen nor talked to Dr. Keel for several days, and because of this, I believe Dr. Keel was assessing if and how we would conduct follow-up with her. She was making a continued effort to treat Amy and offered to prescribe antidepressant drugs. I immediately informed Dr. Keel that Amy would be better when she returned to her regular home environment as an indirect way to let her know that we weren't interested in any more of her recommendations. The attending nurse in the room probably sensed this and began telling me that Amy was not to take any baths because the surgical wounds that still had quite a bit of healing to do. This was when Dr. Keel launched a spirited disagreement with the nurse about Amy's ability to take baths so soon after her surgeries. Dr. Keel disagreed with the nurse, saying that there was no problem for Amy to be able to sit in standing water, but the nurse absolutely opposed it and said that in her experience, no patient with Amy's type of wounds had ever been allowed to sit in standing water so soon after surgery.

Lastly, Dr. Keel says Amy was given a walker for home use, "primarily because she still had some problems with the left knee buckling *from an old injury*", even though it was rather obvious (from the observable swelling and pain) that Amy sustained a more recent injury to this knee while in the hospital. How can Dr. Keel state without any uncertainty that this knee complication was the result of an old injury and not something more recent? It is factual that Amy's leg was injured while she was unconscious and totally in the care of the defendant and hospital staff. It is also factual that the walker was required due to physical injury from the recent surgery (or surgeries), not because of an old injury. Amy's knee was not in an injured condition before she entered the hospital.

These differences may seem minor, but in litigation they could be significant in establishing that the doctor made errors recounting the events. All these inaccuracies that I have raised will have to be examined and weighed against other physician's notes and hospital records. I am confident these will be exposed. Dr. Keel will obviously be given the benefit of the doubt by the court and the jury.

It does seem, however, there may have been a conscious effort by Dr. Keel to cover her bases. When my attorneys reviewed Amy's medical records from Dr. Keel's office (the records from the doctor's practice, not the records from the hospital), it was recognized that every visit was recorded by short, to-the-point handwritten notes. But the January 20xx consultation visit for the hysteroscopy/laparoscopy procedure was a page and a half, single-spaced, type-written record that fabricates a lot of detail discussed that actually never was. According to my attorney, it is so different than any other part of the file it simply sticks out as overtly thorough when compared against the rest of the recorded visits; though our case will not be argued over informed-consent, the truth remains that the actual consultation visit Amy and I had with Dr. Keel was at most, a four-minute, abbreviated version in which the doctor arrived at the appointment 20 minutes late and conducted the consultation hurriedly.

Nevertheless, despite the consultation visit insertion in Dr. Keel's office records, and in spite of errors found in the discharge summary, using the doctor's own summary of Amy's past treatment and hospitalization events was the best way to communicate the clinical version of what happened to Amy. Now, I will summarize the events on that day with my own, personal experience and knowledge of what happened:

Dr. Keel is a specialist in obstetrics and gynecology who, over the course of approximately nine months, diagnosed, treated and performed medical procedures on my wife, Amy. The final procedure Dr. Keel recommended and performed on Amy was an outpatient hysteroscopy with laparoscopy, which took place on March 7th of 20xx. This procedure resulted in severe and life-threatening injuries for Amy and translated into a 16-day hospital stay, six of which were spent in critical care, three of which were spent under life support. The surgery for which Amy was admitted was never performed due to the emergency situation that transpired. During surgery, the doctor severed, tore or damaged the anterior and interior vena cava in my wife's abdomen and other internal injuries that would not be discovered immediately. The damage to the major blood vessels resulted in massive blood loss (2000 cc's or 4.22 pints). To perform emergency vascular repair, her abdomen had to be entered through a major vertical incision made from just below the sternum all the way down to several inches below the navel, approximately twelve inches long. The loss of blood had to be replaced and the situation required a transfusion. A central line through which the transfusion was to be received was placed incorrectly into the subclavian artery by anesthesiologist, Dr. Lister. The blood that Amy received filled her chest rather than enter her blood stream. Amy was rushed back into surgery and given an emergency thoracotomy and repair of the damaged subclavian artery. The thoracotomy resulted in a 12-inch long incision starting at the ribcage just below the right breast, and curving around her right side, ending on her back, just below the right shoulder blade. Postoperatively, three chest tubes were inserted, two on the right and one on the left. The prognosis for Amy was dire and doctors were concerned for organ failure, system failure and possible brain damage. In the ICU, a Swan catheter was attempted to be ran through the left iliac artery, but this tore into and through the artery and eventually had to be run through the right iliac artery. On the morning of March 8th, she was taken back into surgery to repair additional vascular damage to the vena cava, left-iliac artery, and colon. She underwent three major surgeries within a 24-hour period.

Thankfully, Amy survived this shocking series of events. But as if surviving all this wasn't enough, Amy's left knee somehow sustained an impact injury while in or being transported to, between or from one of the surgeries. The hospital staff reported to me twice that my requested x-rays of Amy's swollen knee were normal. A later emergency room visit to Lakeside North Hospital, a different hospital not associated with the one where Amy was injured, revealed that this same knee had been recently fractured. This injury was also confirmed by Dr. Olsen, an orthopedic specialist whom we were referred to by our family physician. Dr. Olsen took his own x-rays and was immediately able to determine the fracture on Amy's patella. While it is possible that this injury was a mistake, there is no question that it occurred during Amy's hospitalization. The medical staff intentionally kept this information from us and in doing so, became negligent in their failure to address Amy's total health; this failure to inform us of the injury hindered our ability to get it properly treated.

Amy's continued medical care wasn't an option, and this led to visits with numerous doctors: Dr. Sanders, our family physician, treated Amy and gave us referrals to Dr. Hanson, a neurologist, Dr. Vickers, a psychologist, Dr. Olsen, an orthopedist who examined Amy and set up treatments for physical therapy three times a week at the McConnell Rehabilitation Clinic, and an assessment referral to Dr. Porter – not necessarily a good doctor in my opinion. Dr. Hanson, the neurologist, would continue to treat Amy, and gave us a referral to Dr. Talbot, a neurosurgeon. Dr. Olsen, who would also be a treating physician for Amy, gave us a referral to Dr. Anderson, a pain management specialist. Amy was also seen by Dr. Smith, an eye doctor, Dr. Gossland, a urologist, and Dr. Brock, a disability doctor for the Social Security Administration. These visits required many trips for MRIs and CT scans.

Through these additional visits, it was discovered that Amy suffered nerve damage in the pelvic area in the left femoral nerve. This was diagnosed as femoral nerve palsy by Dr. Hanson and confirmed by Dr. Talbot. Dr. Hanson also confirmed atrophy of the quadriceps of Amy's left leg. He also diagnosed osteopenia – a precursor to osteoporosis – in the patella of the same leg. Amy was also hit with other physical ailments that simply did not exist prior to the surgeries of March 7th and 8th: constant, ongoing pain; issues with short-term memory retention; degraded motor skills and coordination; irregular sharp pains in the abdomen, sides and lower back; sharp pains in her pelvis during menstrual cycle; soft tissue pain and scarring along the incision wounds of her abdomen, right and left sides and back; frequent headaches ranging from mild to intense; blurred vision in the right eye and a drooping of the right eyelid; but the pain and mental anguish she suffered, accompanied by many sleepless nights and several emergency room visits, can never be fully realized by anyone who didn't experience it personally.

This is the real result of the medical injury she lived through. One might presume that the medical establishment, in seeing this, would flood in to help our cause, acknowledging that their colleagues failed to the highest degree in violating the sacred trust that patients place in their doctors. I don't know about everyone else, but for me to know that I've injured someone, be it accidentally or otherwise, my conscience would propel me to confront the situation in the most honest fashion. In our medical malpractice case, professionals motivated by honesty were far and few and no such rally ever emerged. In fact, all evidence today suggests that both sides have geared up for one long, nasty and personal battle that neither party seems willing to give up any ground.

CHAPTER 21

Building the Case: Larren vs Defendants

The development of the Larren versus Dr. Keel, Dr. Lister & Presbyterian Medical Center malpractice case is a considerable part of our whole story, because in it we discovered firsthand the absolute difficulty of trying to build and maintain a case against all responsible parties. We discovered that the process to pursue these matters legally is a very fragile one; and in light of all the injuries, pain and mental anguish Amy suffered, including the struggle to get our lives back on track from this reeling setback, the burden of trying to put it all together into a comprehensive case to present to a jury, rests on the shoulders of our legal team. This is the primary purpose why I am going into such detail about our case. It so clearly illustrates the point I want to convey regarding the difficulty of litigating a malpractice case, even in one that might seem to satisfy so obviously the key questions medical malpractice firms look to answer before taking on a medical negligence case.

Perhaps the most offensive thing about our medical injury malpractice case is that as a husband, I pride myself on my ability to protect my spouse and family; but in a malpractice case, and certainly in our malpractice case, the damage that was done resulted in extensive physical injuries for Amy, and so a sacred trust was violated. As Amy's prime defender, I was not able to protect her directly while she was alone being treated by the physicians. Honestly, I entrusted them with her care, expecting them to prioritize her medical treatment as if she were a close member of their own family. But once the injury has occurred, it becomes very personal and the only thing one has left is to successfully sue those responsible, forcing them to compensate us for the pain and misery they've caused.

If the most offensive thing about this malpractice case is the breach of trust caused by the injury, then the most *frustrating* thing about pursuing this case is the resistance we get from many in the medical community knowledgeable about the case. The more the defense digs in its heels and resists our effort for proper discovery, the more intense and personal this case becomes to me. Their action registers in my subconscious mind that their opinion of Amy's quality of life as very low and not as important as their own. Sure, they have a right to a defense, but we also have a right to claim the evidence suggests that Amy's injuries were caused by members of the medical establishment. Since those facts are indisputable, then I would think that out of obligation, those close to the situation would come forward voluntarily and provide us with proper honest answers to help Amy recover financially what was taken from her physically. But being things as they are, it is my responsibility to my wife to get this case tried successfully for the highest degree of damages possible. It is, in fact, my personal mission.

Once I signed the Representation Contracts with the attorneys who visited me in the hospital on March 8th, I was committed to pursuing the malpractice case legally. But the official legal contest began when the petition was filed with the court in August that same year. Here is a list summary of how our case is being pursued by our legal firm:

1. Petitions filed with the Court

2. Plaintiff receipt and response of Interrogatories and Production Requests from the Defense legal team of Dr. Keel

3. Amended Petition filed with the Court

4. Additional Plaintiff receipt and response of Interrogatories and Production Requests from the Defense legal team of Dr. Lister and Presbyterian Medical Center

5. Plaintiff Discovery Interviews with Key Hospital Personnel, Treating Physicians, and post-discharge Treating Physicians

6. Plaintiff legal team Depositions obtained of Dr. Milton, Dr. Wales, Dr. Lister and Dr. Edwards

7. Defense legal team Depositions obtained of Amy and Seth Larren

8. Defense legal team Deposition obtained of Plaintiff Expert Witness, Dr. Lee Harren

9. Plaintiff legal team Deposition obtained of primary defendant, Dr. Keel

10. Plaintiff legal team Deposition obtained from the Defense Expert Witness, Dr. Porter

11. Mediation date to be set

12. Pre-trial date to be set

13. Trial date to be set

A petition was filed in court by our attorneys on August 8, 20xx. Originally, XMR Health, Inc., Presbyterian Medical Center, Inc. and Dr. James Lister, were not listed as co-defendants in our case, but as the case moved forward, these defendants eventually were added in an Amended Petition to the court. Presbyterian Medical Center, Inc. and Dr. James Lister are being represented by the same legal firm that is representing Dr. Evelyn Keel.

The original Petition our attorneys filed with the court reads as follows:

Amy Larren and Seth Larren, husband and wife, Plaintiffs, vs. Dr. Evelyn J. Keel, Evelyn J. Keel, M.D., P.C., Dr. Evelyn J. Keel, d/b/a ████████████████████████████, Dr. Evelyn J.

Keel, d/b/a ████████████████████████████████ ,
and ████████████████████████ , Defendants.

PETITION:

COME NOW the Plaintiffs, Amy Larren and Seth Larren, and for
their actions against the Defendants of Dr. Evelyn J. Keel,
Evelyn J. Keel, M.D., P.C., Dr. Evelyn J. Keel d/b/a
████████████████████ , Dr. Evelyn J. Keel, d/b/a ████████
████████████████████████ , and ████████
████████████████████████ , allege and state the following:

1. Amy and Seth Larren are husband and wife.
2. Defendant Evelyn J. Keel is a physician licensed in
    the State of - - -, holding herself out to be a
    specialist in obstetrics and gynecology.
3. At all times relevant to these actions, Defendant
    Keel was acting as an agent and/or employee of
    Defendants Evelyn J. Keel, M.D., P.C., ████████
    ████████████████████ , and ████████████████
    and, as such, Evelyn J. Keel, M.D.,
    P.C., ████████████████████████████ , and ████████
    ████████████████████████████ are responsible and
    liable for the acts of their employee and/or agent
    by reason of the doctrine of *respondeat superior*.
4. On or about March 7th, Defendant Keel performed
    surgeries on Amy.
5. Defendant Keel failed to exercise the ordinary care
    required of a specialist in her field causing severe
    and permanent disfigurement and injuries, lost wages,
    medical expenses and severe physical and mental pain
    and suffering.
6. Defendant Keel's negligence and medical malpractice
    caused injuries and damages to Amy and Seth has lost
    the services, society, comfort and companionship of
    his wife.

7.   Defendant Keel was in exclusive control of the surgical procedures and the instrumentality causing injury and, while under Defendant Keel's care, Amy suffered physical injuries that could not have occurred in the absence of negligence and the doctrine of *res ipsa loquitor* applies.

WHEREFORE Plaintiff's Amy and Seth pray for judgment against said Defendants in an amount in excess of Ten Thousand Dollars for actual damages, mental and emotional pain and suffering, past and future lost wages, past and future medical expenses and such and other relief as the Court may deem just and appropriate.

<u>ATTORNEY LIEN CLAIMED</u>. <u>JURY TRIAL DEMANDED</u>.

Aside from how "lawyerish" the petition might sound, in reading it two terms may jump out at you: *respondeat superior* and *res ipsa loquitor*. Both terms are of Latin origin, and both have distinct legal meaning.

Respondeat superior is a term that means "Let the master answer." This phrase refers to an employer's liability for any actions taken by an employee within the scope of the job. My attorneys named additional defendants on the petition because they were unable to determine exactly which entity employed Dr. Keel at the time she was treating Amy. It is likely that some of the defendants listed will drop off upon proof they are not the responsible parties.

Res ipsa loquitor means "the thing speaks for itself." It is a legal doctrine or rule of evidence that creates a presumption that a defendant acted negligently simply because a harmful accident occurred. The presumption arises only if, (1) the thing that caused the accident was under the defendant's control, (2) the accident could happen only as a result of a careless act, and (3) the plaintiff's behavior did not contribute to the accident.

Res ipsa loquitor is exactly the reason why I feel we have an exceptional case. But even so, it will still be very difficult to successfully try this case without ample preparation, supporting documentation, and skillful presentation of our case. Defense attorneys are very skillful in representing their clients in these types of contests and this will become evident as I cover additional details about our case.

CHAPTER 22

Case Interrogatories

As our case continued to build against responsible parties in our medical malpractice case, Amy and I received INTERROGATORIES through our attorneys from the defense attorneys of Dr. Keel and Northwest Presbyterian Medical Center. These were the first round of information requests that had to be supplied from our legal team. The interrogatories were accompanied with REQUEST FOR PRODUCTION by the defense council. These were received by our attorneys and forwarded to Amy and I for compliance. The request required that we answer them separately and fully in writing, under oath, within 30 days after the mailing of the request, pursuant to (our state's) state law.

As you read through this, keep in mind that this is the defendant counsel trying to get inside our case and request for full disclosure of the foundation off which our case is built. They are essentially asking us to do their work for them.

The questions we had to answer pertained directly to our lawsuit against the parties listed in the petition. I will display the questions from each of the defendants. The Request for Production notification from defendant Dr. Keel reads as follows:

INTERROGATORIES AND REQUESTS FOR
PRODUCTION TO PLAINTIFF

Please take notice that pursuant to Section 3233 of the (State) Discovery Code, you are required to answer separately and fully in writing over our signature and under oath, and serve a copy of the answers upon the undersigned within 30 days after service of the following interrogatories:

INTERROGATORY NO. 1:   State the full name, social security number and date and place of birth of plaintiffs, and whether plaintiffs have ever been known by any other names, and if so, give the other names and state where and when those names were used.

INTERROGATORY NO. 2:   Provide the name and address of all physicians, counselors, therapists or other physical or mental health care providers seen by plaintiff, Amy Larren, for the last 10 years (including drug or alcohol treatment), together with the dates of each visit, reason for each visit and treatment given.

INTERROGATORY NO. 3:   Provide the name and address of all hospitals, clinics, or other health care facilities visited by plaintiff, Amy Larren, for the last ten years (including drug or alcohol treatment), together with the dates of each visit, reason for each visit and treatment given.

INTERROGATORY NO. 4:   Have plaintiffs ever been convicted or pled guilty to a crime other than a routine traffic violation (driving under the influence is not to be considered a routine traffic violation)? If so, list each crime together with the date of the conviction or guilty plea and the court of jurisdiction.

INTERROGATORY NO. 5:   Provide the name and address of all employers of plaintiffs for the last 10 years, together with the dates of employment, description of job duties, salary, and name of immediate supervisor and reason for termination.

INTERROGATORY NO. 6:   Provide the name and address of all persons from whom plaintiffs or their attorneys have secured written or recorded statements, together with the date the statements were secured, whether the person who gave the statement consented to its recordation and the names and addresses of all persons present during its taking.

INTERROGATORY NO. 7:   State whether any physician or other health care provider has stated or implied that any facet of the care given by any defendant was negligent or otherwise below acceptable medical standards. If so, for each provide:

   a.   The name and address of the person making the statement.
   b.   The name and address of the person to whom the statement was made as well as the names and addresses of all persons present during the conversation;
   c.   The date and place the statement was made;
   d.   Set forth fully what was said.

INTERROGATORY NO. 8:   Provide the names and addresses of all health care personnel whom you feel have the opinion that the injuries to plaintiff, Amy Larren, were caused by or worsened by the care or lack of care of any defendant. For each person you list state what you understand their opinion to be.

INTERROGATORY NO. 9:   State whether you believe any medical record on plaintiff, Amy Larren, is false or inaccurate. Specify each entry you disagree with, state what you contend an accurate entry should state and provide the names and addresses of all persons whom you feel support your correction.

INTERROGATORY NO. 10:   State whether you believe any medical record on plaintiff, Amy Larren, was altered or fraudulently created by specifying each entry and for each state all circumstances you rely upon and provide the names and addresses of all persons whom you feel share your opinion.

INTERROGATORY NO. 11:   Provide the name and address of all witnesses whom you believe may testify at the time of trial. For each describe the nature of their testimony and what you understand it will be. In particular, specifically delineate if any witness is being designated as an expert on behalf of plaintiffs.

INTERROGATORY NO. 12:   Provide the names and addresses of all health care personnel whom you feel have the opinion that the defendant or any of them properly managed plaintiff, Amy Larren, and/or complied with acceptable standards of medical care. For each state the basis for this opinion (i.e. personal conversation, conversation with a third party, written correspondence, etc.).

INTERROGATORY NO. 13:   Provide the style and case number of all lawsuits, whether civil or criminal, worker's compensation and bankruptcy claims and divorce proceedings, involving any plaintiff together with the court of jurisdiction. For each suit state whether depositions or other discovery measures were given and set forth the outcome of the case.

INTERROGATORY NO. 14:   State whether plaintiffs have entered into any type of settlement or compromise with any person or entity as a result of the injuries set forth in your Petition. If so, provide the name and address of all persons or entities and state the amount of the settlement.

INTERROGATORY NO. 15:   Have any of the medical expenses which you relate to this lawsuit been satisfied by a payment from the government Medicare/Medicaid program?   If so, set forth the nature and extent of these payments.

INTERROGATORY NO. 16: Fully recite any statement, conversation or behavior by any defendant, nurse or employee of any defendant who you observed or were informed about which you feel to be inappropriate and for each, provide the names and addresses of all present.

INTERROGATORY NO. 17: Was plaintiff, Amy Larren, ever rejected for, or dismissed from, employment for physical or psychological reasons? If so, for each such rejection, state the employer involved, the position or job for which application was made, the condition or reason for the rejection and the date of such rejection.

INTERROGATORY NO. 18: Was plaintiff, Amy Larren, ever rejected for insurance coverage for physical or psychological reasons? If so, for each such rejection, state the insurance company involved, the kinds of insurance coverage for which application was made, whether the coverage applied for was to be under an individual or a group policy, if the coverage was to be under a group policy, the employer or group sponsoring the policy, the condition or reason for the rejection and the date of such rejection.

INTERROGATORY NO. 19: Prior to the injuries described in our Petition, did plaintiff, Amy Larren, have any permanent injury, permanent disability, or preexisting condition, or any hereditary or genetic condition? If so, describe in detail the condition, disability, or injury including, but not limited to, its cause and how it has affected her.

INTERROGATORY NO. 20: State whether you or your attorneys had the medical care and treatment provided by the defendant physicians reviewed by a medical consultant, health care provider or expert witness prior to your filing this action.

INTERROGATORY NO. 21: List all medical expenses which you contend were incurred as a consequence of the alleged negligence of the defendants described in your Petition. As to each, state the amount of such expense, the reason for the expense, and whether the expense has been paid.

INTERROGATORY NO. 22: Plaintiff's Petition makes generalized allegations of negligent or improper conduct by the physician defendants in the care and treatment of plaintiff. Specifically state what you contend the physician defendants you have sued should have done that they did not do or what they did do that should not have been done. Avoid conclusions and specifically itemize the medical tests, techniques or devices you assert should or should not have been utilized.

REQUESTS FOR PRODUCTION OF DOCUMENTS

REQUEST FOR PRODUCTION NO. 1:
Produce copies of any and all medical and pharmacy bills incurred as a result of the injuries which are the subject of the instant action.

REQUEST FOR PRODUCTION NO. 2:
If you are claiming lost wages or earnings as part of your damages herein, produce income tax records, both State and Federal, for the past 5 years, including W-2 statements.

REQUEST FOR PRODUCTION NO. 3:
Produce copies of any exhibit you anticipate utilizing in the trial of this matter.

REQUEST FOR PRODUCTION NO. 4:
Produce copies of any pictures, videotapes, or other illustrations which have been made to depict either Amy Larren's injury or the subject incident.

REQUEST FOR PRODUCTION NO. 5:
Produce copies of all medical records you have secured on Amy Larren.

REQUEST FOR PRODUCTION NO. 6:
Produce any notes, diaries, or other written statements attributable to the plaintiffs or any witness which pertain to the facts of the subject incident or the injuries which plaintiffs contend were incurred as a result of the subject incident.

REQUEST FOR PRODUCTION NO. 7:
Please execute and deliver the Medical Authorization Form attached to these Interrogatories.

REQUEST FOR PRODUCTION NO. 8:
With regard to any allegations of negligence or malpractice contained in your Petition, produce any and all documents, memoranda or reports which substantiate your allegations.

REQUEST FOR PRODUCTION NO. 9:
Produce copies of all written or recorded statements taken by plaintiffs or plaintiff's attorneys of persons knowledgeable of the events in litigation.

REQUEST FOR PRODUCTION NO. 10:
Produce a copy of any report you have secured from a physician or other health care provider concerning the appropriateness of the care given to Amy Larren.

REQUEST FOR PRODUCTION NO. 11:
Produce a copy of any x-rays you or any of your consultants possess concerning Amy Larren.

REQUEST FOR PRODUCTION NO. 12:

Produce copies of all medical literature possessed by you or your attorneys which you believe support your position on any issue in litigation.

Here is The Request for Production notification from defendant Northwest Presbyterian Medical Center. This notification came later than the first, after an Amended Petition was filed with the court, including the Northwest Presbyterian Medical Center and Dr. Lister as additional defendants. Again, read carefully the questions asked and pay careful attention to the thoroughness of the questioning.

INTERROGATORIES TO PLAINTIFF AMY LARREN

Defendant Northwest Presbyterian Medical Center, Inc., propounds the following interrogatories to the plaintiff Amy Larren, requesting she answer the following separately and fully in writing under oath, within 30 days after the mailing of this request, pursuant to the provisions of Okla.Stat.tit. 12, § 3233.

Wherever the words "plaintiff," "you," or "your" appear, or any pronoun referring to the plaintiff, the same shall be taken to refer not only to the plaintiff individually, but also to her attorneys, agents, employees, investigators, representatives, relatives, and any other person who has to the time of answering these interrogatories acquired knowledge of facts in the interest of the plaintiff concerning matters which are the subject of this litigation.

These interrogatories are intended to ascertain information not only in the possession of the plaintiff individually and the other persons named above, but also contained in records and documents in their custody or control or available to them.

Interrogatories which cannot be answered in full shall be answered as completely as possible and incomplete answers shall be accompanied by a specification of the reasons for the incompleteness of the answer, as well as by a statement of whatever knowledge, information, or belief you possess with respect to each unanswered or incompletely answered interrogatory.

These interrogatories shall be deemed continuing pursuant to the provisions of Okla.Stat.tit. 12, § 3226(E) and to require the supplementation of answers if additional information is acquired between the time the answers are served and the time of trial. Such supplementary answers shall be served seasonably, but not later than 30 days after such additional information is acquired.

INTERROGATORIES

INTERROGATORY NO. 1:   State your full name, present address, Social Security number, and date of birth.

INTERROGATORY NO. 2:   If you contend the hospital's *operating room nursing staff* provided you substandard care, identify by full name, description, or job title (or otherwise sufficiently describe so as to permit their identification) the specific operating room hospital employees whom you contend were negligent, and as to each state in detail and with specificity what you contend they should have done but failed to do, or what they did that they should not have done, and identify by full name and address the witnesses (both lay and expert) who will testify on your behalf in support of this allegation.

INTERROGATORY NO. 3:   If you contend the hospital's *recovery room nursing staff* provided you substandard care, identify by full name, description, or job title (or otherwise sufficiently describe so as to permit their identification) the specific recovery room hospital employees whom you contend were negligent, and as to each state in detail and with specificity what you contend they should have done but failed to do, or what they did that they should not have done, and identify by full name and address the witnesses (both lay and expert) who will testify on your behalf in support of this allegation.

INTERROGATORY NO. 4:   If you contend the hospital's agents or employees provided you substandard care, identify by full name, description, or job title (or otherwise sufficiently describe so as to permit their identification) the specific recovery room hospital agents or employees whom you contend were negligent, and as to each state in detail and with specificity what you contend they should have done but failed to do, or what they did that they should not have done, and identify by full name and address the witnesses (both lay and expert) who will testify on your behalf in support of this allegation.

INTERROGATORY NO. 5:   Do you allege, contend or otherwise claim that any of the medical records made or kept by the hospital defendant have been altered, changed, destroyed or in any manner edited?   If so, describe in detail and with particularity any and all such alleged alterations or changes and your reasons for suspecting same.

INTERROGATORY NO. 6:   Did any agent, servant or employee of the hospital defendant make any statement to plaintiff, or which she overheard or otherwise learned of, which may be considered an admission against interest?   If so, state the full name, telephone number and address of each person making such statement and state the content of such statement.

INTERROGATORY NO. 7:   Has any physician or other health care provider made any statement to you or to anyone else indicating that any aspect of the medical care which you received from the hospital defendant fell below acceptable standards for such medical care or was otherwise improper or unwarranted? If so, state the full name and address of each individual making such a statement, when and to whom the statement was made and describe in detail the statement made.

INTERROGATORY NO. 8:   Have you, your attorneys, or anyone on your behalf, taken or obtained a written or recorded statement of any individual purporting to have knowledge of any of the allegations of your Amended Petition? If so, as to each such statement, and as to each such individual, state the identity of the individual whose statement was taken, the identity of the individual taking the statement, the date of the statement, the form of the statement (whether written or recorded) and the verbatim content of the statement, or, alternatively, attach a copy thereof to your answers to these interrogatories. [Note: In answering this interrogatory it is not sufficient to merely claim "work product" status for such statements. If you intend to claim a work product privilege, you must, nevertheless, answer all portions of this interrogatory except that asking the content of the statement.]

INTERROGATORY NO. 9:   Have you or your attorneys consulted with or retained an expert medical witness to testify on your behalf at time of trial? If so, for each such witness, state the expert's full name, address and specialty, the subject matter on which the expert is expected to testify, and state the substance of the facts and opinions to which the expert is expected to testify and a summary of the grounds for each opinion. 12 O.S. §3226(B)(3)(a)(3).

INTERROGATORY NO. 10:   State the full name, address and anticipated testimony of all witnesses who have knowledge of discoverable matters or whom you anticipate calling to testify on your behalf at trial. [Note: For the purposes of answering this interrogatory it is <u>not</u> sufficient to merely state that you have not yet determined who will be called as witnesses. This interrogatory is intended to identify all persons who you reasonably anticipate may be called as witnesses on your behalf even though your attorneys have not made a final determination as to what witnesses will be called.]

INTERROGATORY NO. 11: Describe in detail all injuries which you claim to have suffered as a result of the negligence of the hospital defendant, specifically identifying each type of injury and the location, severity, and harmful effects of each injury. The description of said injuries in your Amended Petition is not sufficiently detailed for an answer to this interrogatory. Include in your answer a description of any mental or emotional injury, as well as physical injuries, for which you are claiming damages.

INTERROGATORY NO. 12: Describe fully and in complete detail all medical and other treatment (including examinations) you have received for the injuries described in your Amended Petition. Include the nature of the treatment, the dates of the treatment, the identity of the physicians or other health care providers providing such treatment, and, if hospitalized, the name and address of the hospital, the dates of hospitalization, whether surgery was performed and, if so, the nature of the surgery performed.

INTERROGATORY NO. 13: Are you claiming any disability to you as a result of the injuries in your Amended Petition? If so, state the nature and extent of the disability, the manner in which it incapacitates you, the date the disability ceased to exist or the estimated future date the disability will cease to exist (if temporary), and the names and addresses of the physicians or other health care providers who have advised you of such disability.

INTERROGATORY NO. 14:   Have you been advised by any physician or other health care provider (or do you otherwise contend) that you will require further medical attention as a consequence of the injuries described in your Amended Petition?   If so, state the full name and address of the physician so advising you and describe in detail the further medical attention that you will require.

INTERROGATORY NO. 15:   Have you lost any earnings as a result of the injuries described in your Amended Petition?   If so, state the reason for such loss of earnings, the dates of missed work, and the amount of any wages, income or earnings lost.

INTERROGATORY NO. 16:   Are you claiming any damages for diminished earning capacity? If so, state the amount of such damages claimed and set forth in detail the calculation by which you have arrived at that figure.

INTERROGATORY NO. 17:   Have you sustained any additional financial losses as a result of the injuries described in your Amended Petition other than those covered by the preceding interrogatories? If so, state the nature and amount of such losses, the date of such losses, and the names and addresses of any person to whom any money so claimed as an additional loss was paid.

REQUESTS FOR PRODUCTION OF DOCUMENTS

REQUEST FOR PRODUCTION NO. 1:
Any and all medical and hospital bills, receipts, invoices, or other documents of whatever nature evidencing the medical expenses allegedly incurred by the plaintiffs.

REQUEST FOR PRODUCTION NO. 2:
Any and all photographs or videotapes showing or relating to the injuries allegedly suffered by Amy Larren.

REQUEST FOR PRODUCTION NO. 3:
Any and all federal or state income tax returns filed by the plaintiffs for the years 1999 through the present, together with any and all records of whatever nature evidencing the plaintiffs' allegations of lost earnings or income.

REQUEST FOR PRODUCTION NO. 4:
Any and all narrative medical reports provided to plaintiffs or their attorneys regarding Amy Larren's medical condition and treatment and the injuries and disabilities which she allegedly suffered by reason of the acts or omissions described in the plaintiffs' Amended Petition.

REQUEST FOR PRODUCTION NO. 5:
Any and all written or recorded statements, audio and/or videotapes, or recordings of any person provided to the plaintiffs or their attorneys regarding Amy Larren's medical condition and treatment and the injuries and disabilities which she allegedly suffered by reason of the acts or omissions described in the Amended Petition, or concerning any of the allegations in the plaintiffs' Amended Petition.

REQUEST FOR PRODUCTION NO. 6:
Any and all notes, diaries, correspondence, or any other written documentation written by or provided to the plaintiffs or their attorneys regarding Amy Larren's medical condition and treatment and the injuries and disabilities which she allegedly suffered by reason of the acts or omissions described in the Amended Petition, or concerning any of the allegations in the plaintiffs' Amended Petition.

REQUEST FOR PRODUCTION NO. 7:
Any and all medical records in the possession of the plaintiffs or their attorneys pertaining to Amy Larren's medical care or treatment *except* those from Northwest Presbyterian Medical Center.

REQUEST FOR PRODUCTION NO. 8:
Any and all exhibits which plaintiffs reasonably anticipate utilizing during any deposition or during the trial of this case.

REQUEST FOR PRODUCTION NO. 9:
Please produce the attached authorization for release of medical records, appropriately executed by Amy Larren.

REQUEST FOR PRODUCTION NO. 10:
Any and all correspondence or written materials provided to plaintiffs by any agent or employee of Northwest Presbyterian Medical Center or NORTHWEST Health.

REQUEST FOR PRODUCTION NO. 11:
Please produce copies of all medical literature possessed by you or your attorneys which you believe support your position on any issue in litigation.

REQUEST FOR PRODUCTION NO. 12:
With respect to each and every expert witnesses you identify or reasonably anticipate calling to testify at the time of trial in this case, please produce the following:

    a.   A current curriculum vitae or resume for the witness, including any publications or presentations;

    b.   The witness' complete file regarding the above-captioned matter, including any and all documents, reports and notes stored on a computer, and any preliminary drafts of any such documents, reports or notes;

    c.   Correspondence to and from your office, including e-mail correspondence;

d.   A list of all cases which the witness has reviewed, or in which the witness has testified (either by deposition or trial) in the last 10 years, including the names of the parties, the case number and court where filed, and the names and locations of counsel for each party.

e.   All records, documents, depositions, articles, or other materials the witness has reviewed or consulted in connection with this case (the witness' copies of such materials, not yours);

f.   Copies of depositions the witness has given in other cases;

g.   Any documents provided to your office by the witness, including but not limited to articles or other literature;

h.   Articles or other literature which the witness referred to in connection with the witness' review and evaluation of this case, or which the witness believes are supportive of his or her opinions;

i.   Billing records, statements, or any other records which would show the amount of time the witness has spent in the review and evaluation of this case, the preparation of a report, consultation with counsel or other experts, or any other work performed on this case.

Whew! What a major dose of detail overkill. Actually, to me, these requests from the defense and the method in which asked illustrates my point exactly as to the tone, what depths and what lengths these guys will go to in effort to construct a strong defense for their clients.

For our case to move forward, Amy and I were obligated to answer the interrogatories truthfully, completely and fully. We returned our answers to our attorneys who reviewed them, filtered them and made motions to object to some or all of the questions based on their right to conduct discovery and retain rights to their work product. The answers we provided in response to the interrogatory questions were thoroughly reviewed by our legal team to prevent the defense from knowing every angle of our case prior to trial.

Still, I asked Amy to review questions 2 – 5 from the second interrogatory questions and answer them again for me so I could print the answers in this book. The reason for doing this is to show how we've interpreted these questions and to again communicate the tone of how this case is shaping up. I have reprinted the questions for better interpretation. The following are her responses to the second series of interrogatories:

INTERROGATORY NO. 2: If you contend the hospital's *operating room nursing staff* provided you substandard care, identify by full name, description, or job title (or otherwise sufficiently describe so as to permit their identification) the specific operating room hospital employees whom you contend were negligent, and as to each state in detail and with specificity what you contend they should have done but failed to do, or what they did that they should not have done, and identify by full name and address the witnesses (both lay and expert) who will testify on your behalf in support of this allegation.

PLAINTIFF RESPONSE: I was completely unconscious and therefore cannot provide the information requested for this interrogatory. No family member or individual protecting my interest was present in the hospital's operating room during my presence there, so it is unlikely any person can provide this information on my behalf. I will instead default to my right through our attorneys to pursue discovery in efforts to determine applicable negligent parties in this setting.

INTERROGATORY NO. 3: If you contend the hospital's *recovery room nursing staff* provided you substandard care, identify by full name, description, or job title (or otherwise sufficiently describe so as to permit their identification) the specific recovery room hospital employees whom you contend were negligent, and as to each state in detail and with specificity what you contend they should have done but failed to do, or what they did that they should not have done, and identify by full name and address the witnesses (both lay and expert) who will testify on your behalf in support of this allegation.

PLAINTIFF RESPONSE: Again, I was completely unconscious and therefore cannot provide the information requested for this interrogatory. No family member or individual protecting my interest was present in the hospital's recovery room during my presence there, so it is unlikely any person can provide this information on my behalf. I will instead default to my right through our attorneys to pursue discovery in efforts to determine applicable negligent parties in this setting.

INTERROGATORY NO. 4:   If you contend the hospital's agents or employees provided you substandard care, identify by full name, description, or job title (or otherwise sufficiently describe so as to permit their identification) the specific recovery room hospital agents or employees whom you contend were negligent, and as to each state in detail and with specificity what you contend they should have done but failed to do, or what they did that they should not have done, and identify by full name and address the witnesses (both lay and expert) who will testify on your behalf in support of this allegation.

PLAINTIFF RESPONSE: I contend the hospital's agents/employees provided substandard care based on the fact that my knee was injured while I was unconscious and the hospital's staff not only failed to address this complaint, but they also intentionally kept knowledge of the injury from me, my spouse and my family. I complained of pain in my knee and my husband, noticing the ample swelling on the knee, requested a knee x-ray be taken. My husband witnessed the x-ray tech taking three separate pictures of this knee and the results of these pictures were never provided until requested by my husband. He was told by the x-ray tech that the results were "negative." Not satisfied with this answer my husband later asked an ICU nurse about the results and was provided the exact same answer. On April 1, 20xx, an emergency room visit to the Lakeside North Hospital obtained an x-ray of my knee and was able to determine from one picture that the knee was recently fractured. This explained why my knee was swollen and why there was pain in my leg. I further contend that the hospital's agents/employees provided substandard care based on the fact that blood was left in my hair and it became matted. For days, the hospital staff made absolutely no effort to clean or remove the blood and clots from my hair, so my sisters came in to wash it, but the matting was so bad that much of my hair came out during the washing and the blood damaged my hair to the degree where it eventually had to be cut. It has taken years to get my hair back to its current level of health. And after my transfer from the ICU, nurses assigned to my care allowed me to fall on two separate occasions during ambulatory exercises, left me on a bedpan for more than an hour and took half-hours to respond to my call light. Being a former CNA, I know these practices are substandard for a hospital in this city. Other matters resulting in injury during my surgeries and nerve damage may have occurred by hospital agents or employees, and my attorney's discovery process may identify this and other instances to fully satisfy this question.

INTERROGATORY NO. 5: Do you allege, contend or otherwise claim that any of the medical records made or kept by the hospital defendant have been altered, changed, destroyed or in any manner edited? If so, describe in detail and with particularity any and all such alleged alterations or changes and your reasons for suspecting same.

PLAINTIFF RESPONSE: I am not knowledgeable enough about all the documentation of my medical records to claim that any part of my records were destroyed or altered. Because I have no knowledge of everything done to me by any potential defendant(s), I cannot confirm nor exclude the possibility that such changes of these records were made, although I do have concerns about ambiguity on the discharge summary and operative reports as prepared by the primary defendant.

As our case progresses, no doubt there will be plenty of discussion regarding Amy's many injuries and how they occurred, but the truth remains that we may never know fully what happened and how certain injuries occurred. The information coming forward is slow and the knee injury is a perfect example of how we will never fully know the cause of some of Amy's injuries. There's no denying the existence of the leg injury, but so far, no amount of probing has determined how it was damaged, and no one has come forward to offer suggestions as to how it may have been damaged. It isn't enough to prove that the leg was damaged; there has to be evidence to suggest how. Agents and employees of the hospital value their jobs too much to help us with this; so as it turns out, there may be no claim for damages on this injury simply because we cannot determine how it happened.

Continuing to build our case, our attorneys obtained records and conducted discovery interviews with Dr. Sanders (Family doctor), Dr. Bennett (from the University ER), Dr. Hanson (Neurologist), Dr. Olsen (Orthopedist), Dr. Anderson (Pain Management Specialist), Dr. Talbot (Neurosurgeon), Dr. Vickers (psychologist) and gynecologists Dr. Porter and Dr. Reysa. These are doctors who either assessed Amy or treated her since the March 20xx hospitalization. These interviews were conducted to help our legal team gauge which doctors might be candidates to strengthen our case and possibly present as witnesses, though it is my belief that the strongest support for our case comes from the medical records obtained from these doctors. The records themselves confirm the depth of Amy's injuries and the difficulty in trying to treat them.

Next, our legal team interviewed again and took depositions from Dr. Wales (the vascular surgeon who performed the second emergency surgery on Amy), Dr. Milton (the vascular surgeon who performed the first emergency surgery on Amy and the third surgery the morning of March 8th, 20xx), Dr. Lister (the anesthesiologist who inserted the central line and caused the injury to Amy's subclavian artery) and Dr. Edwards (the internal specialist who was consulted to coordinate Amy's recovery during hospitalization). These depositions took place over the course of several weeks and probably didn't occur in the order that I listed the physicians.

It wasn't long after the first round of depositions that our legal team dismissed Dr. Lister from the case. It was determined through expert consultation that there simply was not enough evidence to keep him listed as a defendant, even though he had a role in injuring Amy. Dr. Lister has since retired from medicine and with the loss of him as a defendant I felt to some degree that our case had suffered a major blow before it was even fully put together. It is my hope that justice still prevails to compensate Amy for her agony and suffering.

CHAPTER 23

Deposition: Amy Larren

Eventually, the time came for the defense to obtain depositions from Amy and me. Scheduling problems caused multiple postponements, but the final date set for our depositions was November 1, 20xx. We were scheduled to arrive at our attorneys' office at 8:30 a.m. and the parties were to meet in the conference room. Present at the deposition was our attorney, Steve, and two attorneys from the same firm representing the defendants Dr. Keel and Northwest Presbyterian Medical Center. Mr. K. Grant was the attorney defending Dr. Keel and Ms. S. Short was the attorney representing Presbyterian Hospital.

During a deposition there are formalities that are covered, such as making sure the person answering questions understands they need to provide clear, verbal responses. It was decided beforehand that Amy would be deposed first. I was allowed to remain in the conference room and listen as she was deposed. It was one of the toughest things I've ever had to sit through. I want to share just a few portions of our deposition transcripts, beginning with Amy's, to provide an insight into the defense strategy of our opponents. The information printed here does not contain every question asked during the deposition and not every answer to the question is provided here either. But there is sufficient information to get a feel for the unanswered variables of the case. Like me, you may marvel at some of the questions.

Direct Examination of Amy Larren by Defense Counsel, Mr. K. Grant:

Grant: What is your maiden name?

Amy: _ _ _ _ _.

Grant: What is your Social Security number?

Amy: _ _ _ _ _ _.

Grant: And your date of birth?

Amy: _ _ _ _.

Grant: Ever applied for a different Social Security number?

Amy: No.

Grant: Are you currently employed?

Amy: No.

Grant: When was the last time you were employed?

Amy: 20xx, at _ _ _ _ _.

Grant: _ _ _ _ _ was your last employer?

Amy: Yes.

Grant: What was your job title?

Amy: _ _ _ _ _ _.

Grant: Have you applied for work since 20xx?

Amy: No.

Grant: Why not? Is there a reason you haven't?

Amy: My leg injury.

Grant: Any other reason, other than your leg injury, which has prevented you from applying for employment?

Amy: General pain.

Grant: And what leg has been injured?

Amy: My left.

Grant: Have you applied for any disability because of your left leg injury?

Amy: Yes.

Grant: When was that?

Amy: 20xx, several weeks after my discharge from the hospital.

Grant: What happened with that disability claim?

Amy: We were on it for a short while; then we decided to go ahead and get off of it.

Grant: You made a claim for SSI based on your left leg injury?

Amy: Yes.

Grant: Was there any other reason for the claim for SSI, other than your left leg injury?

Amy: I was in a lot of pain, pretty much all over.

Grant: Any other reason other than your left leg injury and you were in a lot of pain all over?

Amy: No.

Grant: The current source of income for the household would be from Seth's job?

Amy: Yes.

Grant: Any other sources of income at this time?

Amy: No.

Grant: Since 20xx, other than your husband's employment and that short period of time you received SSI, did you have any other sources of income at that time?

Amy: No.

Grant: Your son – what's his birthday?

Amy: _ _ _ _ _.

Grant: Who treated you during this pregnancy?

Amy: Dr. Reysa.

Grant: Did you like Dr. Reysa?

Amy: Yes.

Grant: Consider him to be a good physician?

Amy: Yes.

Grant: And where was your delivery?

Amy: University Hospital.

Grant: Have you continued seeing Dr. Reysa since the birth of your son?

Amy: Yes.

Grant: He is your obstetrician-gynecologist?

Amy: Yes.

Grant: Did you see – well, have you sought treatment from any other OB/GYN other than Dr. Reysa?

Amy: No.

Grant: I saw from the medical records you saw at one point a Dr. David Porter.

Amy: Yes.

Grant: Do you remember how many visits you had with Dr. Porter?

Amy: _ _ _ _ _.

Grant: Do you recall why you were treated with Dr. Porter?

Amy: I received a referral from Dr. Sanders.

Grant: Do you know why Dr. Sanders gave you a referral to Dr. Porter?

Amy: I don't remember; I think it was for a checkup.

Grant: How many times did you treat with Dr. Porter?

Steve: Object. You've already asked that once.

Grant: Did you like Dr. Porter?

Amy: No.

Grant: Why not?

Amy: I didn't like his bedside manner.

Grant: What about his bedside manner didn't you like?

Amy: It was just the way he talked to me and stuff... His attitude was hostile.

Grant: What did he say to you?

Amy: _ _ _ _.

Grant: So, because of his body language and his attitude, you didn't care for Dr. Porter?

Amy: No.

Grant: So, it wasn't - - sounds like anyway - - and correct me if I'm wrong – it wasn't really something Dr. Porter said, it was the way he said it and the way he acted. Would that be fair?

Grant: Do you today still experience pain in your lower back and left leg?

Amy: Yes, I do.

Grant: How often do you experience that pain?

Amy: Frequently. But nonstop after my discharge from the hospital for at least two months.

Grant: On a good day, do you have pain in your back?

Amy: I do.

Grant: What sort of activities will cause you to have pain in your back and left leg?

Amy: Lifting, sitting up for long periods of time, going up and down stairs, squatting…

Grant: Any other activities you notice that have caused you pain - -

Amy: Walking for long periods of time, bending down on my knees, riding in a car for a long period of time. Bending over to give my son a bath hurts me a lot.

Grant: And when did you first start experiencing pain in your back and left leg?

Amy: … when I woke up from surgery. I can't remember what day I woke up. I do remember the pain.

Grant: And that's where you remember the pain, when you woke up from surgery, was in your back and left leg?

Amy: The left leg mostly. The back started after I got up moving around.

Grant: Have you sought treatment from a physical therapist for this pain in your back or your left leg?

Amy: I have.

Grant: Did the therapist discharge you from therapy, or did you just decide not to go any longer, or how did that occur?

Amy: They discharged me and gave me strengthening exercises to do at home.

Grant: And what sort of exercises did they tell you to do at home?

Grant: And how often did they want you to do those at home?

Grant: Do you do it there in your home, or do you go to a gym to work out?

Amy: At home.

Grant: Do you keep a record of how often you do those exercises at home?

Amy: No.

Grant: When you were pregnant and seeing Dr. Reysa, did this pain in your leg and back increase during the pregnancy?

Amy: Yes. It did.

Grant: Did you complain to Dr. Reysa about the pain increasing?

Amy: Yes.

Grant: And how long were you on bed rest pursuant to Dr. Reysa's instructions?

Amy: Pretty much the whole pregnancy.

Grant: So, you don't recall a period of time during your pregnancy where the pain wasn't present?

Amy: Right.

Grant: Would it be safe to say that on all of your visits to see Dr. Reysa during the time you were pregnant, you complained to him about this pain in your back and leg?

Amy: Yes.

Grant: When did you first seek treatment with Dr. Evelyn Keel?

Amy: It was in 20xx.

Grant: And why were you treating with Dr. Keel?

Amy: Pregnancy. OB-GYN, all that stuff.

Grant: How did you end up treating with Dr. Keel?

Amy: We found her name on our list of insurance providers.

Grant: Did you know her from any of the other physicians on that list?

Amy: No.

Grant: Was her office close to your residence at that time?

Amy: Yes.

Grant: Had any of your friends or relatives ever treated with Dr. Keel?

Amy: No.

Grant: You said you were pregnant at the time you first saw her?

Grant: How many times did you see Dr. Keel there in her office before the March 20xx hospitalization?

Amy: I don' remember exactly.

Grant: Were there several visits?

Amy: Yes.

Grant: During those visits, did you find Dr. Keel to be nice and polite?

Amy: Yes.

Grant: Did she answer the questions that you had for her?

Amy: Some of them, yes.

Grant: Okay. Was there ever a question that you had for her that she didn't answer?

Amy: Not that I recall.

Grant: Would your husband accompany you on your visits to see Dr. Keel there in her office?

Amy: Yes.

Grant: During those visits in which he would go with you, would he be in the room at the time you're seeing Dr. Keel?

Amy: Yes.

Grant: The office staff that Dr. Keel had, did you find them also to be nice and polite and professional?

Amy: Yes.

Grant: Did it appear to you as if Dr. Keel took her time when she was examining you and explaining to you what was occurring during your pregnancy?

Amy: During the pregnancy? Yes.

Grant: What prompted your hospitalization in March of 20xx?

Amy: She said that I needed to have a surgery performed since I have had miscarriages. I don't remember very much of that conversation, though.

Grant: Was your husband present at the time you and Dr. Keel are discussing this surgery?

Amy: Yes.

Grant: Did she give you any documents, pamphlets, handouts on the type of surgery that you were going to have in March of 20xx?

Amy: No. Not that I remember.

Grant: Did Dr. Keel speak with you about the risks of having this surgery?

Amy: It was a brief conversation. She said there's very little risk, and she's done this procedure a thousand times. She said there's nothing really to worry about.

Grant: And what surgery was she going to perform in March of 20xx?

Amy: Laparoscopy.

Grant: And this conversation that you had with Dr. Keel would have been over 3 years ago by now, right?

Amy: Yes.

Grant: So, there were things said that you're not able to recall. Is that fair?

Steve: Object to the form.

Grant: What you do recall is that she told you there was very little risk?

Amy: Right.

Grant: And that she had performed this procedure, what, a thousand times?

Amy: A thousand times.

Grant: A hundred?

Amy: About a thousand times.

Grant: And as you sit here today now, some 3 ½ years later, you're not able to recall everything Dr. Keel told you about that surgery, are you?

Amy: Right. I just remember (what I've told you) about the risks.

Grant: And in fact, would it be fair to say you're not able to recall all the risks she told you about that surgery?

Grant: Were you still curious, after she told you there was very little risk, as to what those very little risks were?

Amy: Not much, because ...

Grant: Did you know of anyone that had had this type of surgery before?

Amy: No.

Grant: Did Dr. Keel explain to you why she was recommending surgery?

Amy: Yes.

Grant: Why was that?

Amy: She did an HSG. She said she thought she saw a septum.

Grant: And what is an HSG, as you understand it?

Amy: They inject dye into the uterus to view it with equipment.

Grant: And Dr. Keel I think you said mentioned something and there might be a septum?

Amy: Yes.

Grant: And those - - as you understand it, those were the reasons she was recommending the laparoscopic procedure?

Amy: Right.

Grant: Had you had any difficulty with the HSG procedure she did a couple months prior to that?

Amy: I was bleeding really heavy after (the procedure).

Grant: Any other problems with the HSG procedure?

Amy: I was told that there was a miscarriage involved.

Grant: Any other problems?

Amy: Not that I recall.

Grant: What about during the time the HSG is being performed, did you have any problems?

Amy: It was really painful.

Steve: Can we take a break?

[Short break at 10:31 a.m. Resumed at 10:37 a.m.]

Grant: We were just starting to talk about your hospitalization at Presbyterian in March of 20xx. You already told me you recall waking up from surgery and having pain in your left leg.

Amy: And all over -

Grant: All over. Do you recall any of the other events there at the hospital during your hospitalization?

Amy: Just the pain -

Grant: Anything else you're able to recall for us?

Amy: Just not liking being in there, my wanting to go home.

Grant: Sure. Do you recall conversations with physicians?

Amy: I don't remember any of those.

Grant: What about conversations with family members?

Amy: I don't remember any of those.

Grant: Would it be fair to say that everything you've learned about what occurred there at the hospital, Presbyterian, in March of 20xx, you've learned through conversations either with family members or with your attorney?

Amy: Pretty much, yes.

Grant: So you don't have any independent recollection of those events, other than what you've already told me about you being in pain?

Amy: Right.

Grant: Questions like how many other physicians treated you, what they treated you for; you wouldn't have any information about that?

Amy: No, I wouldn't.

Grant: Same with respect to the nurses there at the hospital, how many times they were in and out of your room, you wouldn't have any information about that?

Amy: No, I wouldn't.

Grant: Before March of 20xx, did you have problems with your back or left leg?

Amy: No.

Grant: Before March of 20xx, were you ever restricted in any of the work that you did because of problems either with your back or your left leg?

Amy: No.

Grant: Before March of 20xx, did you ever have a problem with your left leg or left knee?

Amy: No.

Grant: Before March of 20xx, did you ever seek medical treatment for problems with your left knee or lower back?

Amy: The left knee I do remember. I'm sorry – left knee ...

Grant: You sought medical treatment for problems with your left knee before March 20xx?

Amy: Yes.

Grant: Did you ever seek medical treatment for problems with your lower back before March 20xx?

Amy: No.

Grant: Why were you seeking treatment for problems with your left knee before March 20xx?

Amy: I hurt it on the job. I sprained it. Hyperextended it.

Grant: And where were you working at the time you sprained your left knee?

Amy: I believe I was working for Home Health...

Grant: How did you sprain your left knee?

Amy: Helping lift a patient to a wheelchair.

Grant: And did you seek medical treatment for that sprain of your left knee?

Amy: Yes.

Grant: Who treated you?

Grant: Was it at a hospital, physician's office?

Amy: A hospital.

Grant: Did you go to the emergency department?

Amy: Yes.

Grant: How many times did you go to the emergency department?

Amy: Just once.

Grant: But your work wasn't restricted because of this sprain to your left knee?

Amy: Restricted, yes, it was.

Grant: You told me about a previous injury to your left knee, you sprained it while you were working, and you went to some emergency room for treatment. Is that the only time you sought treatment for your left knee sprain?

Amy: Yes.

Grant: Okay. How did they treat your left knee sprain at that time? Did they give you a brace?

Amy: A brace... an immobilizer...

Grant: Did you go through any sort of physical therapy?

Amy: No.

Grant: How long did you have to wear this brace?

Amy: For about a week or two.

Grant: And did the brace help?

Amy: Yes.

Grant: So, after a week or two, you took the brace off and were able to carry on with your job?

Amy: Yes.

Grant: No other problems with that left knee after that point in time but before March 20xx?

Amy: No.

Grant: Who have you treated with since March of 20xx, for these problems with your left leg and back?

Grant: Did you see Dr. Keel after your hospitalization at Presbyterian?

Amy: No, I didn't.

Grant: Is there a particular reason why you didn't see Dr. Keel after that hospitalization?

Amy: Because of the stuff that happened in the hospital.

Grant: You were aware that at the time of your discharge from Presbyterian, there was a follow-up appointment?

Amy: Yes.

Grant: And you chose not to attend that follow-up appointment?

Amy: Right.

Grant: What about what happened in the hospital made you not follow up with Dr. Keel?

Grant: Did you at any point in time ask Dr. Keel what happened during your surgery?

Amy: No, I didn't.

Grant: Do you know if any of your family asked Dr. Keel what happened during the surgery?

Amy: I don't (know). I'm sure they did, though.

Grant: Do you know how many surgeries you had during your stay at Baptist in March of 20xx?

Amy: I was told three on one day and one on another day.

Grant: Do you know why it was necessary for you to have that many surgeries?

Amy: To fix what (Dr. Keel) did.

Grant: We've been produced some photographs in this lawsuit - - or several of those. Do you have any idea who took those photos?

Amy: No, I don't.

Grant: Do you have any idea why those photographs were taken? Were they taken for purposes of this lawsuit?

Amy: I presume; Yes.

Grant: Do you have any idea when an attorney was first contacted about filing a lawsuit in this case?

Amy: I don't (know) – I do know it was while I was in the hospital.

Grant: So, you understood – or you now understand that the attorney was contacted while you were still hospitalized at Northwest Presbyterian Medical Center?

Amy: Yes.

Grant: Were you aware that correspondence had been sent from your attorney to Dr. Keel in Presbyterian Hospital during your hospitalization?

Amy: I was not aware.

Grant: One of your previous employers was _ _ _ Nursing Home?

Amy: Right.

Grant: And you worked there I believe as a nurse aide?

Amy: Yes.

Grant: And I believe you told us that, in answering some questions for us, you worked there from February of 20xx, through March of 20xx?

Amy: Yes.

Grant: And why did you leave _ _ _ Nursing Home?

Amy: I was moving to another side of the city.

Grant: They didn't ask you to leave?

Amy: No.

Grant: And you weren't terminated?

Amy: No.

Grant: During the time you worked for _ _ _ Nursing Home as a certified nurse aide, did you have any on-the-job injuries?

Amy: No. I can't remember. The only one I remember is once getting bit by a patient.

Grant: The only on-the-job injury that you recall during your employment with (_ _ _ Nursing Home) was being bit by a patient one time?

Amy: Right. That's all I remember.

Grant: I'll hand you now - - we can mark this if we need to. This is from your employment file with _ _ _ Nursing Home, dated February 20xx. It says that while you were lifting a resident into bed, you hurt your back on February 16th of 20xx, and that you are complaining of ongoing pain in your lower back. Do you remember hurting your back during your employment with _ _ _ Nursing Home?

Amy: I can't remember...

Grant: In fact, this is a medical record from _ _ _ Medical Center.

Amy: I remember that.

Grant: You remember going to _ _ _ Medical Center for treatment?

Amy: I remember there, but - - I'm trying to...

Grant: And this is your name up at the top?

Amy: Right.

Grant: Amy, how do you pronounce your (maiden) last name?

Amy: _ _ _ _ _ _

Grant: And it says here that to treat these complaints of pain in your lower back, that you're going to be given a large cold pack and started on some physical therapy.

Amy: Okay.

Grant: Wasn't that their plan for you?

Amy: I don't really remember. I really don't.

Grant: That's what it says under Treatment Plan of the record; right?

Amy: Right.

Grant: And did you complete this course of physical therapy for these complaints of pain in your lower back?

Amy: I don't remember.

Grant: Reviewing that record, does that refresh your memory of sustaining an injury to your lower back during your employment with _ _ _ Nursing Home?

Amy: No, it doesn't.

Grant: I take it you're not going to claim that record is inaccurate?

Amy: Right.

Grant: This is a follow-up record. You see you returned to _ _ _ Medical Center again, because of pain in your back, and you also were "complaining of some pain in her left knee, but this is unrelated to the current injury." Do you see where they've written that in your medical record?

Amy: Yes.

Grant: What problems were you having with your left knee at that time?

Amy: I don't remember...

Grant: It says that the problems you expressed to them in your left knee, they were unrelated to the current injury - - that injury to your back. How had you injured your left knee before February of 20xx?

Amy: That must have been when I sprained it that first time.

Grant: When you sprained it when you were working for _ _ _ Home Health care?

Amy: Yes.

Grant: And what period of time were you employed with _ _ _?

Steve: Objection. You asked that and she's answered already. Go ahead, answer it again.

Grant: Was it before your employment with _ _ _?

Amy: Yes.

Grant: In fact, down here in the Plan, it says "We will continue the physical therapy and modify the work restrictions." Is that what they have underneath their plan?

Amy: Yes.

Grant: Do you know what sort of modifications they were making to your work restrictions?

Amy: I don't remember.

Grant: Do you know what type of restrictions had been placed on your work prior to this visit with _ _ _ Medical Center?

Amy: I don't remember.

Grant: Did you sustain any other injury while working on the Job, other than injury to your left knee that you told us about, an injury to your lower back that we've seen from these medical records?

Amy: Just what I have now.

Grant: But as far as other on-the-job injuries -

Amy: No.

Grant: - you didn't have any others besides the left knee sprain you told us about and the lower back pain we saw from the medical records?

Amy: Right.

Grant: So, after February of 20xx, you did not continue to complain of pain in your lower back. Is that true?

Amy: I did probably - maybe to the doctors.

Grant: So, after February of 20xx, when we saw you complaining of pain, to the folks there at _ _ _ Medical Center, you continued to complain of pain in your lower back?

Amy: Yes.

Grant: And you saw physicians for that pain in your lower back?

Amy: No.

Grant: You just continued to have that pain?

Amy: Yes.

Grant: In fact, wasn't that one of the reasons you left _ _ _ Nursing Home?

Amy: No.

Grant: So, your back problems had nothing to do with your leaving _ _ _ Nursing Home?

Amy: Right.

Grant: The physicians that you currently see for complaints of pain in your left leg and lower back, have they told you what causes that pain?

Amy: The causes? They just said it will heal in time...

Grant: With additional time, this pain will resolve? Yes?

Amy: Right.

Grant: To your knowledge, no one has ever told you what causes you to have pain in your left leg and lower back. Is that fair?

Amy: Right.

Grant: And you do agree that prior to March of 20xx, you had complained of pain in your left knee and lower back? True?

Steve: Object to the form. You can answer, Amy.

Amy: My left knee and back, yes.

Grant: After your release from Northwest Presbyterian Medical Center and you started noticing this pain in your left leg, were you ever treated - - or did the physicians ever treat that with a brace, an immobilizer, anything of that nature?

Amy: Yes.

Grant: And how long did you wear the brace?

Grant: Do you know who prescribed that brace?

Amy: I don't remember, exactly-

Grant: Do you remember leaving Presbyterian Hospital with a brace?

Amy: I don't remember.

Grant: And you would agree that if you were given a brace or immobilizer to wear on your leg, you should follow those instructions and wear it, right?

Amy: Right.

Grant: And you did, during your treatment, follow the instructions given to you by your physicians?

Amy: Right.

Steve: Object to the form.

Grant: And if you didn't follow those instructions, you understood it would be a little bit more difficult for you to heal properly?

Steve: I'll object again to the form of the question. You can answer it.

Amy: Yes.

Grant: Before the deposition began, your attorney gave us some tax return information. This is your tax return for the year of 20xx?

Amy: Yes.

Grant: And your signature appears at the bottom of page 2 of that return, does it not?

Amy: Yes.

Grant: And you list your occupation as a student?

Amy: Yes.

Grant: Was that the period you were seeking this training at _ _ _ Business School?

Amy: Yes.

Grant: Have you been involved in any other litigation besides this lawsuit?

Amy: No.

Grant: No one has ever sued you before?

Amy: No.

Grant: And you've not sued anyone else other than Dr. Keel and Northwest Presbyterian Medical Center?

Amy: Right.

Grant: Have you ever had to file for bankruptcy?

Amy: No.

Grant: Have you ever filed a Workers' Compensation claim?

Amy: No.

Grant: Who's babysitting your son today?

Amy: My mom.

Grant: I take it you stay at home with him during the day when your husband is at work?

Amy: Yes.

Grant: And you're able to care for him?

Amy: Yes.

Grant: You said he's seven months old?

Amy: Yes.

Grant: Who is his pediatrician?

Grant: Any plans on having more children?

Grant: I'll pass the witness.

At this point, Direct Examination begins by defense counsel, Ms. S. Short, representing Presbyterian Hospital. Here are some of the questions asked by Ms. Short during this deposition. Again, these questions do not include every single question asked because of space limitations. Because of these same limitations, I will not record any of the responses.

Short: *Mrs. Larren, my name is S_ _ _ Short. We met earlier this morning. And I will tell you that I represent Presbyterian Hospital. Some of my questions may come from that perspective.*

At the outset, you told us several of your prior residences, as well as your current residence. Have all of those been apartments on the second floor?

Is there any reason that you and your husband prefer a second-floor apartment?

Is there a specialty or a type of physician that you recall seeing since you were discharged from the hospital in March of 20xx, but you can't remember the individual's name?

I looked through some bills that — medical bills that were provided to me this morning, and I see, for example, in here a medical bill from the _ _ _ _ _ Eye Institute. And I think the physician's name is Hester, H-e-s-t-e-r. Why did you see Dr. Hester?

Do you still have droopiness in the lid of your right eye?

Do you still have blurriness?

Did Dr. Hester give you any indication as to the cause of either the droopiness or the blurry vision?

Have you seen anyone other than Dr. Hester for eye problems?

Did Dr. Hester prescribe any kind of treatment, be it medication or something else, because of the eye problems?

Do you wear glasses? You don't have contacts in this morning, do you?

Do you continue – well, strike that. Let me ask you this. It's my impression, Mrs. Larren, that you have had some improvement with both the droopiness in your lid and the blurring, is that right?

Have doctors told you to anticipate any kind of continued improvement, be is slight or otherwise?

Are you hopeful that you will continue to have some kind of improvement with your lid or your blurry vision?

Can you tell me when you first noticed the blurry vision?

Did you have it while you were still hospitalized? The blurry vision, that is?

When did you first notice having a droopy lid?

Other than perhaps a cosmetic change or result, has the droopy eyelid caused you any problems? Obviously an eyelid that droops may be appreciable to other people; true? And there may be some cosmetic effect from that. Other than the fact that there may be a cosmetic effect, have you had any other kind of adverse effect from the fact that your right eyelid droops?

Do you mind if I look at those photographs for just a second? Mrs. Larren, let me hand you a couple of photographs. I'm handing you four from this stack of photographs that have been taken. And just for the record, I will describe them *as pictures taken of your face from a frontal view. Can you tell me the purpose of these four photographs?*

Do you know when these four photographs were taken?

Can you give me any kind of time frame as to when the photographs were taken, albeit I understand you can't give me a date?

Do you believe these photographs were taken when your eyelid was at its worst?

Can you tell me who took those pictures?

Are you aware of any other photographs that were taken to represent your eyelid droop?

Also, in this stack of photographs, there were obviously quite a few photographs taken while you were still on a ventilator or the respirator. And I would assume you had no appreciation that the photographs were taken?

Okay. Some of these photographs, for example, that were taken while you were on the ventilator, I'm assuming because of your medical condition you didn't understand or realize that anybody was taking pictures?

I apologize if you told us this. Do you know who took the photographs taken while you were still hospitalized?

Let me hand you a photograph that was taken while you were still hospitalized at Northwest Presbyterian Medical Center. It is undated, but there is the back of a female in the photograph. Can you identify that individual for me?

Who is (Belinda) Copeland?

Is she your age or your mother's contemporary?

Would it be a fair and accurate summation of your testimony that you don't have any memory of the events that took place at Presbyterian Hospital in March of 20xx, other than recalling waking up and being in pain?

So, you couldn't tell me anything about the nurses that were involved in your case, any discussions you had with the nurses or therapists, those sorts of things?

Do you believe all of your family members were able to visit you while you were hospitalized at Baptist?

Let me hand you one of the photographs taken while you were at Presbyterian Hospital, and it looks like it represents perhaps a chest tube insertion site or some type of small incision under your arm. Can you tell me who is helping take the photographs? Look at those hands and see if you can recognize those.

Do you have any idea, Mrs. Larren, what your out-of-pocket medical expenses have been, associated with your hospitalization at Baptist in March of 20xx?

Do you know if you or your husband have received any kind of mail or telephone calls from bill collectors with respect to any of the medical expenses associated with your hospitalization?

Have you ever received any phone calls from Dr. Keel's office?

What about from Presbyterian Hospital?

Have you received any kind of mailings from Dr. Keel's office with respect to payment?

What about Presbyterian Hospital? Have you received any kind of mailings from Presbyterian Hospital with respect to payment?

Do you have any idea how much blood was utilized, given to you?

There were (some) depositions taken in this case prior to yours today. Have you read those deposition transcripts?

Have you looked at any notes made by any family members while you were hospitalized?

Obviously, the photographs were taken while you were hospitalized and at various times thereafter. Are you aware of any videotapes that have been taken since you were discharged from the hospital?

You said that your friend – or your mother's friend, Belinda, who saw you while you were hospitalized, they were friends through church? What church was that?

Did you discuss your care or the care you received at Northwest Presbyterian Medical Center, with Dr. Porter?

Did you discuss with Dr. Porter at all any of the events that occurred during your hospitalization at Baptist?

But you don't recall asking Dr. Porter about Dr. Keel's care and the surgeries that you had?

Do you recall Dr. Porter making any statements to you about the care you received at Northwest Presbyterian Medical Center from Dr. Keel?

This concludes Amy's portion of the deposition. I must add that during the deposition, Amy was nervous and answered some of the questions inaccurately – not intentionally, but out of nervousness. She didn't relax, nor take deep breaths, nor take the time to properly listen to the questions and think through the answers. She was so tense that she downplayed many of her answers, kept them short. I think she was intimidated by the attorneys' method and/or tone of questioning. And, she had suffered through some short-term memory loss surrounding the time she regained consciousness after the botched surgery and even past her discharge from the hospital. Her recollection was not fully intact and her answers didn't really hurt our case, but was a missed opportunity to significantly help our case.

Regardless, prior to our depositions, Amy and I were coached by our attorney to provide only "yes" or "no" answers as often as possible, as to not "lock" ourselves into any specific testimony where we might be susceptible to deviate from during cross-examination at trial. Adhering to this is very difficult because human nature entices one to respond to these questions defensively, and it's hard to do that without providing more information than what is being asked. But it is good advice to provide simple answers to only the question being asked because it may save you from the defense attorneys shredding you on the witness stand during trial.

In Mr. Grant's questioning of Amy, there were some answers to the questions that demand elaboration, and here they are:

Q.   What happened with that claim for disability?

A.   We were on it for a while; then we decided to go ahead and get off of it.

The claim for disability benefits was denied, based on records the SSA received from Dr. Porter, Dr. Anderson, Northwest Presbyterian Medical Center, and Dr. Brock, the SSA's examining physician. The SSA's provided response, "We have determined your condition was not disabling on any date through 12/31/20xx, when you were last insured for disability benefits. In deciding this, we considered the medical records, your statements, and how your condition affected your ability to work." Did they really? If there was any time I felt as if Amy and I were being dumped on, this was it. It is also a strong reason as to why I vote republican. In my observation, government does not provide much help to those who really qualify for it and anytime it does provide help, it is difficult to access and very conditional.

Even though Amy was denied disability benefits, she eventually received SSI benefits in November of 20xx, but the benefits were not retroactive to the date of her injuries even though the injuries forced her to resign from work. And these SSI benefits were contingent upon my income and regular appointments with the SSA. If I made less than a certain amount in a calendar month, the monthly benefit payment would be around $220.00, but if I made above a certain amount in a calendar month, then the monthly benefit would drop to about $30.00. This was tough to gage and too conditional to rely on, so we concluded that I would be better off getting a second job and doing away with the SSI benefits altogether. We contacted the SSA to inform them of our decision and were told we could not discontinue the benefits with a simple phone call. It was difficult to get the benefits started and still difficult to end them, so we intentionally missed Amy's next scheduled SSA appointment, which by default cancelled the benefits.

Q. *And you would agree that if you were given a brace or immobilizer to wear on your leg, you should follow those instructions and wear it, right? And you did, during your treatment, follow the instructions given to you by your physicians? And if you didn't follow those instructions, you understood it would be a little bit more difficult for you to heal properly?*

Amy answered these questions as if she wore the immobilizer per the doctor's instructions, but she failed to remember that she couldn't wear the immobilizer because the entire surface of her leg was painful. She couldn't allow anything to touch it. Muscle tone in her leg degenerated and the damage to the nerve tissue in the femoral nerve emitted pain all over her leg. Also, the bone started to lose density, but these issues couldn't be addressed medically until repair or restoration of the femoral nerve. This leg caused her many sleepless nights, and the pain was such that she wanted it amputated. Because of these reasons, she couldn't wear the immobilizer. She couldn't tolerate the pressure and pain it caused her to have it on her leg.

Q. *Did you like Dr. Porter?*

A. *No.*

Q. *Why not?*

A. *Didn't like his bedside manner.*

Q. *What about his bedside manner didn't you like?*

A. *It was just the way he talked to me and stuff.*

Q. *What did he say to you?*

Q. *So, because of his body language and his attitude, you didn't care for Dr. Porter?*

244

A. No.

Q. So, it wasn't - - sounds like anyway - - and correct me if I'm wrong – it
wasn't really something Dr. Porter said, it was the way he said it and the
way he acted. Would that be fair?

There were reasons beyond his bedside manner and attitude that we didn't care for
Dr. Porter. During his examination of Amy, he opined that her injuries were a *common and
accepted* risk of having a laparoscopy procedure done. This, and his inability to be
empathetic, helped us forge our opinion of him. It amazes me how anyone can think so
highly of themselves that they are incapable of extending compassion to an innocent
individual injured by one of his colleagues. To think that this guy still treats women within
the metro area is a personally disturbing thought.

Q. Would it be safe to say that on all of your visits to see Dr. Reysa during the
time you were pregnant, you complained to him about this pain in your
back and leg?

During pregnancy, Amy had multiple visits to University Hospital until the birth of our
son in March of 20xx. Dr. Reysa recorded those adhesions on her uterus, suspect from the
injuries of her hospitalization in March of 20xx, was the reason the pregnancy was so much
trouble. Amy's pregnancy which resulted in many more hospital visits which likely would
not have been necessary if she hadn't sustained medical injuries while hospitalized. The
pain in her back and leg were compounded by the pregnancy weight gain. Dr. Reysa, being
the extraordinary doctor that he is, recommended total bed rest and steered away from
overzealous procedures.

Q. During those visits, did you find Dr. Keel to be nice and polite?

A. Yes.

Q. Did she answer the questions that you had for her?

A. Some of them, yes.

Q. *Okay. Was there ever a question that you had for her that she didn't answer?*

Well, obviously Dr. Keel wasn't too forthcoming with *all* the risks. She overplayed Amy's need for the surgery and downplayed the risks by emphasizing her own experience in performing the procedure. How could we ask the proper questions if we weren't properly informed in the first place? We didn't know enough to be more concerned about potential risks.

Q. *Do you recall watching a video on the type of surgery that she was going to perform?*

A. *No.*

Q. *Did she give you any documents, pamphlets, handouts on the type of surgery that you were going to have in March of 20xx?*

A. *No. Not that I remember.*

At no time prior to Amy's surgery (or afterwards) did the doctor or any of her staff provide us documents, pamphlets, handouts, nor did we watch any video. In fact, it surprised us to learn that they show a video to patients before allowing them to go through this procedure.

Q. *We were just starting to talk about your hospitalization at Baptist in March of 20xx. You already told me you recall waking up from surgery and having pain in your left leg.*

A. *And all over -*

This portion of the deposition illustrates how sly some (if not most or all) malpractice defense attorneys attempt to minimize the suffering of malpractice victims. His question was an intentional effort to lock Amy into a testimony isolating her pain to her left leg, when the fact of the matter is, she suffered pain everywhere there was an incision wound, chest tube wound, internal pain from the injuries and post-operative pain, in addition to her left leg – which endured an impact injury in the hospital, even though Mr. Grant tries his best to structure a scenario where Amy's leg was somehow re-injured by a strain that occurred over a year before Amy's hospitalization. Someone should have informed Mr. Grant that the evidence supported a recent impact injury on Amy's knee over his "mysterious" theory that the leg would somehow re-injure itself while Amy was unconscious. This question angered me – and though I am not a violent person, I found myself wishing I could take a hammer to his knee.

Q.   Would it be fair to say that everything you've learned about what occurred there at the hospital, Baptist, in March of 20xx, you've learned through conversations either with family members or with your attorney?

A.   Yes.

Q.   So you don't have any independent recollection of those events, other than what you've already told me about you being in pain?

A.   Right.

Q.   Questions like how many other physicians treated you, what they treated you for, you wouldn't have any information about that?

A.   No, I wouldn't.

Q.   Same with respect to the nurses there at the hospital, how many times they were in and out of your room, you wouldn't have any information about that?

Again, this questioning doesn't take into account the amount of discomfort, pain and agony Amy was In. In case Mr. Grant isn't aware, when someone is in excruciating pain, they aren't concerned about what other people happen to be talking about at the time. A person in severe pain is not concentrating on how many physicians treated them, how many times nurses entered in and out of their room or anything like that; they are concerned about getting relief. This question angered Amy; in her anger she forgot that there were some things that she remembered with respect to being left on a bedpan for over an hour, call-light responses from the nurses that took over 30 minutes, falling on two separate occasions in the hospital while trying to ambulate, and the incident involving Dr.

Milton where he held her against the bed to force down the NG tube. But with respect to what Mr. Grant was asking, Amy wasn't counting physicians or nurses, nor was she trying to collect information to help our attorneys. She had other things to be concerned about, like how well she was going to be able to function once released from the hospital.

I mentioned earlier how the defense checked into Amy's and my personal past and background, trying to dig up dirt for purposes of assaulting our character during trial. If the defense had any real doubt that Amy was fabricating any of her injuries, is there any question they would have hired a private investigator to track us and gather evidence exposing this? We have no way of knowing that they didn't try, but it stands to reason that their absence of referring to any kind of material proof contradicting Amy's injury claims inadvertently substantiates that they know that her injuries are real.

CHAPTER 24

Deposition: Seth Larren

The break at 10:31 called by our attorney, Steve, during Amy's deposition, was requested by me because I found myself getting angrier and angrier at the questioning. I went to the restroom and washed my face with cold water, after punching a hole in the sheetrock with my fist. If I could have turned into the Hulk right then and there, half of all downtown in our city would have been destroyed. The questioning by Mr. Grant appeared to be from the standpoint that all of this was Amy's fault because we decided to take legal action. Amy was being drilled only because the doctor, in her failure to competently perform the surgical procedure, determined she was going to fight this case.

My deposition ran longer than Amy's, as I was asked more questions and had better recollection of events than she. And though I was allowed to sit through her deposition, Amy would be absent from mine; the stress that it put on her made it unnecessary for her to sit through my testimony. I was geared up and ready to get to it – or through it. Again, this deposition is not printed in its entirety, although the most significant questions are covered. The answers provided are from both the actual deposition and revised answers after my review of the deposition transcript.

Grant: (After asking for a complete list of everyone who visited Amy in the hospital, from our respective families, friends, members from church, etc.) Did you or anyone else to your knowledge, ever keep any notes during the time your wife was hospitalized at Northwest Presbyterian Medical Center?

Seth: Not during the time she was hospitalized.

Grant: Did you at any time make any notes while your wife was hospitalized at Northwest Presbyterian Medical Center?

Seth: No.

Grant: Are you aware of anyone that made any notes at the time she was in the hospital at Northwest Presbyterian Medical Center?

Seth: Not other than the doctors.

Grant: At any time, have you ever had a chance to review the notes that the doctors made about your wife's care at PMC?

Seth: Just the discharge summary and operative reports; outside of that, I haven't had a chance to review.

Grant: So, you're not aware of any family member, friend, relative that kept any notes while your wife was hospitalized at PMC?

Seth: No.

Grant: Are you aware of anyone who has prepared notes about your wife's stay at PMC, after she was discharged home?

Steve: Object, to the extent that that might be privileged information if I've asked him to do something. So notwithstanding (To Seth) that I've asked you to do or someone else in my office has asked you to do.

Seth: No.

Grant: So, you're not aware of any relative (or) friend that prepared notes regarding your wife's stay at Presbyterian, after she was discharged?

Seth: No.

Grant: Have you at any time ever prepared any notes about her stay at PMC?

Steve: Again, I'm going to object to the extent –

Grant: He can answer if he's prepared notes. And if it's for you, that's fine.

Steve: Go ahead.

Seth: Yes, I have prepared notes.

Grant: When did you first begin preparing those notes?

Seth: Not really until after she got home.

Grant: You said, "not really." That kind of makes me uneasy.

Seth: I had not begun making any notes before she arrived home from the hospital.

Grant: And why did you make those notes?

Seth: Pretty much they were just personal notes. It was a Day Planner calendar, and it was just a log of some different events that I thought were –

Grant: Were you requested by anyone to keep notes?

Seth: No. I was not requested by anyone to keep notes.

Grant: Do you still have those notes?

Seth: No.

Grant: Where are they?

Seth: We have moved since then and in the process of moving we purged a lot of different stuff. And we still have some purging to do with regards to stuff that we've accumulated, but – we don't collect a lot of stuff. We like to keep the house free of clutter.

Grant: Understood. Did you make any entries on a computer, about your wife's stay there at the hospital, at any time?

Seth: Just in relation to responding to interrogatories.

Grant: Other than that, no other entries on a computer?

Seth: No.

Grant: So, the notes that you did have about your wife's hospitalization at Presbyterian have been discarded or lost or something?

Seth: Correct.

Grant: Your wife was hospitalized at Baptist from March 7th to March 22nd, 20xx. Is that consistent with your memory?

Seth: That is.

Grant: And when did you first contact an attorney about filing a lawsuit?

Seth: I didn't contact an attorney. One was contacted on my behalf. I didn't know that Amy was going to survive. The doctors weren't expecting her to survive. I wasn't even thinking along those lines. My brother-in-law, who happened to be in town during this period, arrived at the hospital and tried to discuss this with me; today I'm kind of glad that he was there to help me think along those lines.

Grant: What brother-in-law?

Seth: Chris Resar.

Grant: So, your brother-in-law, Chris Resar, first brought up the subject of filing a lawsuit?

Seth: He asked me if I wanted him to connect with attorneys on behalf of Amy and myself.

Grant: How long had he been at the hospital before he brought this up with you?

Seth: ...I called him on the day that Amy was in the hospital, when everything turned south, and I called him in order to get her on a prayer list, because at that point no one expected her to survive.

Grant: So, your brother-in-law, Chris Resar, was in town on March 7, 20xx?

Seth: That's correct.

Grant: And because you and he spoke on the phone frequently, he was aware Amy would be entering the hospital that day for surgery?

Seth: That's correct.

Grant: And at some point during the day on March 7th, you called Chris to tell him to place your wife on the prayer list?

Seth: Yes.

Grant: And was It at that - - I'm trying to figure out what point in time did Mr. Resar suggest to you that finding an attorney may be a good thing to do?

Seth: It was much later on that day. ...he and my sister showed up at the hospital later on that evening, of the 7th.

Grant: And that's when he first brought up the subject of filing a lawsuit or contacting a lawyer?

Seth: Yes.

Grant: And did you make any efforts at that time to contact a lawyer?

Seth: I had not.

Grant: Did Chris make any efforts to contact a lawyer on your behalf?

Seth: He and I had a conversation and he essentially said to me that it wasn't his place to tell me what to do, but he told me that I might want to consider getting attorneys involved, to protect my and Amy's interests. He said (Amy) deserved better treatment than what she received, and I should probably start thinking along those lines (to hire an attorney).

Grant: This would have been a conversation you had with Mr. Resar before or after your wife's second surgery?

Seth: It was before the final surgery on the morning of the 8th, but after all the surgeries that took place on the 7th.

Grant: What efforts, if any, did Mr. Resar take on your behalf to secure an attorney?

Seth: He told me it would be no trouble for him to contact a person from his congregation who had a daughter that lives in (our city) that was an attorney and told me to tell him yea or nay, and that he'd make the call.

Grant: And you gave him permission to make the call?

Seth: Not immediately, but before he left that night. I was reluctant to address the issue because I didn't want to appear to be an opportunist, and I didn't want to detract from Amy's care. I wanted the doctor's attention to be on getting her healed and felt that (hiring attorneys) would be a distraction. So initially, I tried to sidestep it, but he was persistent. And like I said, I'm glad that he was there.

Grant: So, before Mr. Resar leaves the evening of March 7th, he has your permission to contact the member of his church who has relatives that are attorneys here in (this city)?

Seth: That's correct.

Grant: And is it your understanding that Mr. Resar placed those calls?

Seth: Yes.

Grant: And how do you know that?

Seth: Well it's obvious: the attorneys contacted me early in the morning on the 8th.

Grant: And is that the attorneys from this office?

Seth: Yes.

Grant: At any point in time did you mention to the physicians or the nurses that were taking care of your wife that you had contacted an attorney?

Seth: No.

Grant: And again, I think you mentioned a little earlier you really didn't want that to be public knowledge, distract them from taking care of your wife?

Seth: Right.

Grant: The phone call you received from attorneys in this office on March 8th, 20xx, was that a result of a call they placed to your wife's room at Presbyterian?

Seth: No. No call was never – that I'm aware of, ever placed to my wife's room.

Grant: Would have been through your cell phone?

Seth: There was a call that was placed through the hospital phone, and from that particular phone call was how I got in touch with the attorneys here.

Grant: She left you with a number that you then called?

Seth: No, she didn't leave me with a number at all. After that conversation, she arrived at the hospital and then the (other) attorneys arrived at the hospital.

Grant: So, there were attorneys from this office in the hospital on March 8th, 20xx?

Seth: That is correct.

Grant: How many visits did they make to PMC during the time your wife was receiving treatment there?

Seth: 2 to 3.

Grant: We've got a stack of photographs over there. Did you take any of those photographs?

Seth: Yes, I did.

Grant: Did any of the attorneys from this office take any of those photographs?

Seth: Yes.

Grant: If we were to go through the pile, could you tell us which photographs the attorneys from this office took?

Seth: I cannot.

Grant: If we were to go through the pile, could you tell us which photographs you took?

Seth: Not with any certainty. I could guess, but I wasn't the only one taking them. Amy's mother took a few.

Grant: Amy's mother, you and attorneys from this office took photographs; anyone else?

Seth: Crystal, Amy's older sister.

Grant: Photographs that Amy's mom and sister took; do you know which of those photographs (they took)?

Seth: No, I don't.

Grant: Were any of these photographs made prior to the attorneys from this office coming to the hospital on March 8th, 20xx?

Seth: No.

Grant: Do you know how your wife ended up treating with Dr. Keel?

Seth: It was a joint decision between her and me. We identified a doctor that was on our insurance list and one that was close by where we lived.

Grant: Were you looking for a certain specialty?

Seth: We were looking for a specialist, yes, for OB/GYN.

Grant: And why were you looking for that specialty?

Seth: Well, we just wanted a good doctor, and it was our perception that a board-certified specialist was a good doctor.

Grant: But was your wife having some problems at the time that she needed treatment from a specialist?

Seth: No, not at all.

Grant: Had she been treating with any other physicians, family physicians, prior to that time, to your knowledge.

Seth: No.

Grant: Did you accompany your wife on any of her visits she made to see Dr. Keel?

Seth: Yes.

Grant: How many times would you go with her?

Seth: Just about every time, with the exception I'd say of maybe about two.

Grant: Did any other family members go with your wife on those other occasions which you did not attend?

Seth: Her mother.

Grant: Was her mother also present when you were there?

Seth: On one of the visits – or at least one of the visits, but yes.

Grant: You sat through your wife's deposition this morning; true?

Seth: I did.

Grant: And do you agree with her assessment of Dr. Keel during those office visits?

Steve: Object to the form. Go ahead and answer.

Grant: And if you don't recall, let me just repeat the questions for you. Did you, during your interactions with Dr. Keel, find her to be nice, polite, and professional?

Seth: Yes.

Grant: Did she seem to take time, spend time with your wife, examining her and making sure she understood what her condition was?

Seth: Initially she spent a lot of time with us, and we liked her. And even after - - well, we continued to see her. In hindsight, I believe there was probably a few visits where we felt she could have spent a little more time with us, but our main assessment of her was that we liked her and we trusted her.

Grant: And you said she initially spent a lot of time with you. Did that change during the course of your treatment with Dr. Keel?

Seth: Well, it's questionable. Maybe it's just perception, but – I could bring up a particular situation – but the way I perceived it was she's a doctor, doctors are busy; they get called on emergencies. And that was how I rationalized those questionable moments. But for the most part, during our visits there was nothing that really concerned me.

Grant: Nothing you saw from Dr. Keel or her staff concerned you to the point where you needed to go back to that list of physicians and find another one for your wife?

Seth: Right.

Grant: And I take it you were aware that Dr. Keel had planned surgery for your wife to take place at PMC on March 7th, 20xx?

Seth: Yes.

Grant: Nothing you saw from Dr. Keel, her behavior with your wife, the time she spent with your wife, caused you enough concern to question her performing surgery on your wife on March 7th, 20xx?

Seth: No.

Grant: Would it be fair to say that you felt comfortable with Dr. Keel performing surgery on your wife March 7th, 20xx?

Seth: Yes.

Grant: Were you present at any time when Dr. Keel was discussing the surgery she was going to be performing in March 20xx?

Seth: Yes. We did have a consultation visit at which I was present.

Grant: And what do you recall from that conversation?

Seth: I recall from the conversation that she did describe a little bit about the procedure, and she did say that there were some risks, but she qualified that with, "I've performed this procedure many times and I never encountered any of the risks."

Grant: Anything else?

Seth: And as far as how she explained the surgery, she described briefly how they would go in through a small incision in the abdominal wall to view the uterus from the topside so that while they were through the pelvis at the other end, they're not in there trying to blade a septum blindly. She said by viewing the uterus from the topside through a small incision in the abdomen minimizes the risk.

Grant: Anything else?

Seth: That's it.

Grant: Would it be fair to say that Dr. Keel's description to you of the surgery she was going to perform was discussed in more detail, it's just that with the passage of time you're not able to recall all of those details?

Seth: It's not fair to say that at all. I do remember that particular morning of the consultation the appointment was scheduled at 10:00 – and I remember this because at the time I was working at - - -, and my sales territories were Las Vegas and Los Angeles, which is a Pacific time zone. So, I was required to be at work at 10:30, and I would leave work at about 7:00 at night. I had made arrangements to be at work slightly late that day for the appointment, and we arrived at Dr. Keel's office just before 10:00. Dr. Keel was running late and at this particular appointment, she was – you know, there were times before this where she was late to an appointment with us, but at this particular one she was later than any of the prior times, to the tune of at least 20 minutes late. And I kept looking at my watch because I took my job seriously and wanted to be there to make my solicitations. When you're getting paid commission, you want to be at work to try and make your sales. But on that particular day, she was about 20 minutes late. And when she finally arrived, she spent about 4 minutes – not quite 5 minutes – with us. And the gist of that consultation was, "we know that Amy can take anesthesia well, she's had the D&C's before in the past; we know she has no drug allergies." Then basically she just confirmed the date of the surgery.

Grant: Did you ask Dr. Keel why she was late that morning?

Seth: No, I didn't ask her why she was late.

Grant: Was it your understanding that Dr. Keel delivers babies?

Seth: Yes, I do understand that she delivers babies, and kind of had an idea that maybe she was doing something else with another patient. I know that at one point in the past, prior to that consultation meeting that she had arrived at University Hospital for us on an emergency basis – the second D&C that occurred in December. So, you know, it wasn't too much of a concern of mine that she was late that day – (albeit later than any of the other times).

Grant: All right. Was there anyone else present with you that day which surgery was discussed, other than you and your wife?

Seth: Just me and my wife.

Grant: Do you know what time you were able to make it in to work that day?

Seth: ...?...

Grant: Okay, and you said during this visit is when Dr. Keel explained to you a little about the surgery she's going to perform?

Seth: Right.

Grant: And she told you that there were risks associated with this particular surgery; right?

Seth: Again, she didn't go into detail at all about the risks. She said she had never encountered any of the risks and added, "I've performed this procedure many times." She didn't put any particular number on how many times she had done the procedure. I believe where Amy got confused with the number was a statement by another doctor who placed a number on something. (Dr. Keel) said she performed the procedure many times and she had not encountered any of the risks.

Grant: Did you understand how she was going to make an incision through the abdomen so she could look at the uterus?

Seth: I understood the purpose of the last – it was going to be a small incision so that there wouldn't be a big scar that would be a reminder of the surgery. So yes, I did understand how they were going through a small incision in the abdominal wall.

Grant: Did she discuss with you the fact this was going to be a surgery performed with a laparoscope – it's going to be a laparoscopic procedure?

Seth: Yes.

Grant: And did she tell you how that would be performed?

Seth: Not in any detail, other than what I've already told you.

Grant: Certainly, if you wanted to spend more time with Dr. Keel that day, you could have?

Seth: Possibly, yes.

Grant: If you had any questions that, in your mind, were not answered by your visit with Dr. Keel that day, you would have asked them at that time, true?

Seth: Right.

Grant: Same thing with your wife. If she had any questions that, in her mind, were unanswered, she would have asked that of Dr. Keel that day?

Seth: Yes.

Grant: And your memory of that conversation, Dr. Keel tells you that she has performed this procedure many times, versus what your wife said, thousands of times?

Seth: Yes. It wasn't a hundred times, it wasn't a thousand times – it was "many" times.

Grant: And you said you believe your wife's statement that Dr. Keel had performed (the procedure) a thousand times was based on a conversation with another doctor? What other doctor was she talking to?

Seth: More recently she went to see a urology doctor that she was referred to by Dr. Reysa. And when we went to this appointment, he said, "I understand that you had some issues in the past with medical treatment and doctors," to which Amy acknowledged. And he says, "Yeah, with laparoscopic surgeries, you generally want the doctor to have performed at least a thousand of those before you trust them to perform one on you." And we weren't even aware that he knew about it. I guess that probably the referring physician, Dr. Reysa, informed him that Amy was really apprehensive about seeing doctors, and maybe he discussed with this doctor why she was apprehensive.

Grant: Do you know how many Dr. Keel had performed before March 20xx?

Seth: No. Why should I know that?

Grant: Who was this doctor and how you spell his name?

Grant: Was this doctor aware of the fact that your wife had received treatment from Dr. Keel, or was he aware that your wife had filed a lawsuit against Dr. Keel?

Seth: I don't know any of that. There was nothing he said that led me to believe that he knew there was a lawsuit or the name of the doctor involved in Amy's treatment.

Grant: So, he didn't reference Dr. Keel's name at all during your conversation?

Seth: Not at all.

Grant: Getting back to the discussion you and your wife had with Dr. Keel immediately before surgery, you were told by Dr. Keel that she has performed this procedure before – "many times" I think was your words.

Seth: Yes; her words.

Grant: And that she had never encountered any of the risks?

Seth: Right.

Grant: Did you or your wife at any point ask Dr. Keel, "Well, Dr. Keel, what are those risks of surgery?"

Seth: No, we didn't – but that doesn't absolve her from full disclosure-

Grant: And is it your testimony that at no time did Dr. Keel tell you what those risks of surgery-

Seth: That is my testimony.

Grant: Did you receive any documentation from Dr. Keel about the surgery?

Seth: Honestly, I don't – you know, I heard you ask Amy that during her testimony and, like her, I don't recall ever seeing any literature and certainly no video.

Grant: Did you receive any paperwork, documents, which told you the type of surgery that was going to be performed, and the risks of the surgery?

Seth: I don't recall ever receiving any of that, and if I had to wager money on it, I'd say no, we didn't receive any printed literature.

Grant: You don't recall Amy signing any paperwork in the office that day, saying that she had reviewed some documents concerning surgery, which discusses the procedure and the risks of the procedure?

Seth: She signed nothing on that day; she signed multiple papers the day of the surgery.

Grant: So I take it when you left the office that day, you didn't have a question about what risks associated with this surgery Dr. Keel was going to perform.

Seth: Right. I wasn't knowledgeable enough to really understand that there were multiple risks. But at the time we left, we were consciously satisfied that we had all the information we needed, and I had no other concerns.

Grant: Did Dr. Keel speak with you about other types of surgeries that could be performed to address your wife's problems?

Seth: No. As a matter of fact, I was surprised that there were other surgeries – and this was well after the (surgery had already taken place) – but that there were other surgeries that could have been done in place of this one. We learned this from Dr. Reysa, but we hadn't covered any of them with Dr. Keel.

Grant: So you just remember Dr. Keel discussing the laparoscopic procedure?

Seth: Right. We decided to go with this, based on her recommendation, and we weren't offered any other alternative.

Grant: So you only remember her – Dr. Keel – discussing with you the laparoscopic procedure, and none of the other procedures?

Seth: No; just the laparoscopic and hysteroscopy.

Grant: You remember after the (December 20xx) HSG procedure, probably during, (Amy) was in a lot of pain?

Seth: Yes. I wasn't in the room where the procedure was being performed, but after the procedure Dr. Keel came out and told me it was a painful experience for Amy.

Grant: And I'm sure Dr. Keel told you at that time what she found from the HSG?

Seth: I remember she said she saw what appeared to be a cyst in Amy's uterus, in addition to what she saw to be a uterine septum. At that point she said she was going to give us a referral to a specialist whose name I don't remember. Because she said there was a cyst, I didn't even question it because I knew Amy's sister in the past had a bout with cervix cancer, so there was no reason for me to believe that Dr. Keel was inaccurate in describing what she saw as a uterine cyst.

Grant: And she gave you a referral to a specialist?

Seth: Yes, but we never saw him.

Grant: Why is that?

Seth: Because of an emergency room visit that happened in December following the HSG, where Amy ended up seeing Dr. Keel again during that emergency room visit. As a result of that, Keel and I determined that it wasn't necessary for (Amy) to see the specialist.

Grant: You say Keel and you determined that.

Seth: During the conversation I had with Dr. Keel on that day after the emergency D&C, it was agreed between us that – and I was the one who brought it up. I asked her, "this being the case, it wouldn't be necessary for Amy to see this specialist that you were talking of in our last office visit?" And Dr. Keel agreed.

Grant: You said, "...this being the case." What was the case?

Seth: Amy had to have an emergency D&C during that emergency room visit. Prior to
            that was the HSG test done only days earlier. We (Amy & I) were surprised to
            learn that the emergency room physician diagnosed Amy as miscarrying, and
            we were surprised because Dr. Keel's office told us that Amy wasn't pregnant
            after we consulted her to provide us that confirmation. So, Dr. Keel was called
            in to perform the emergency D&C and she came in and performed it. After the
            procedure Dr. Keel and I talked and I asked her if it were possible that the cyst
            she believed she saw during the HSG was a fertilized egg, to which she replied
            that it was possible. Then she commented that it could have been residual
            tissue from the prior D&C. She apologized for the situation and said that had
            she known that Amy was pregnant, she would not have performed the HSG.

Grant: This was the conversation you were having with Dr. Keel at University; this was
            after the second D&C procedure, is that right?

Seth: That is correct.

Grant: Dr. Keel had previously performed a D&C procedure on Amy, right?

Seth: Yes.

Grant: And that was also accomplished there at University?

Seth: Yes.

Grant: And what was your understanding of why the first D&C procedure was
            necessary?

Seth: Well, the answer to that is rather obvious – don't you think?

Grant: And it's your memory the HSG procedure occurred in between the two D&C
            procedures?

Seth: Yes; only days before the second one.

Grant: After the second D&C procedure, did your wife continue to have problems?

Steve: Object to the form of the question.

Grant: Well, let me ask it this way. When you were talking to Dr. Keel after that second D&C procedure, was it your understanding that she was going to perform additional surgery beyond that?

Seth: Well, our discussion at University after the second D&C ended with Dr. Keel asking, "Are you and Amy scheduled to see me?" Amy and I weren't practicing any family planning and we weren't intent on trying to have a child right away. I mean, Amy got pregnant, she miscarried; she got pregnant again and then had an HSG after the doctor failed to confirm the pregnancy. And so, some of these problems can be attributed to Dr. Keel before the laparoscopic surgery happened, but this was the hand we were dealt and we were too far into our treatment path with Dr. Keel to turn back now. So yes, it was understood between Amy, Dr. Keel and I that Amy would have the laparoscopy done.

Grant: Okay. I think I heard you say that you and Amy, at that point anyway, you weren't actively planning on having a family at that time?

Seth: Right.

Grant: Did you accompany your wife when she saw Dr. David Porter?

Seth: I took her to the office, and I sat in the waiting room while she saw Dr. Porter.

Grant: Did she see Dr. Porter before or after (Amy's) March 20xx surgery?

Seth: After.

Grant: Had you returned to full-time work before Amy was released from the hospital?

Seth: Yes, I had.

Grant: Do you recall how many days you had worked full-time before her discharge?

Seth: Four or five days.

Grant: And you mentioned before that, you were working part-time?

Seth: ...three or four days working partial-days.

Grant: I take it you drove your wife to PMC that day, March 7th, 20xx?

Seth: Yes.

Grant: Before surgery, did you see or have a conversation with Dr. Keel?

Seth: Not between the time we had the consultation visit and the surgery.

Grant: When you arrived at PMC, how did you know where to go?

Seth: The floor receptionist.

Grant: Did you complete any of the admitting paperwork?

Seth: Amy filled it out, and I signed as appropriate.

Grant: Do you recall what sort of discussions were going on between the nurse and Amy at that time?

Seth: I don't.

Grant: Then at some point is Amy taken to a holding area prior to surgery?

Seth: Right.

Grant: Are you present with her up until the time she was wheeled into the operating room?

Seth: Yes. I remained with her until they wheeled her off.

Grant: And at no time prior to the surgery did you see Dr. Keel?

Seth: Briefly, just a minute or two before they took Amy away for surgery.

Grant: Was she there talking with Amy?

Seth: Not only Amy, but there was small conversation along the line of "how are you today," and, "are you comfortable?"

Grant: Are there any family members present at that time?

Seth: No.

Grant: And Dr. Keel comes in, speaks with Amy for a second, and then she - -

Seth: She leaves, and the other personnel come and take (Amy) away.

Grant: Then your next contact with Dr. Keel or any other physician about Amy's surgery would have been when?

Seth: A long while after they took her away.

Grant: You're still at the hospital by yourself?

Seth: Right.

Grant: What's the first information you remember receiving about her surgery?

Seth: A phone call into the waiting room on the surgery floor. A female voice on the phone told me there was a complication with Amy's surgery and that I would personally get additional information from Dr. Keel.

Grant: Do you know who the female voice was on the other end?

Seth: No, I don't.

Grant: Did she explain to you what sort of complication Dr. Keel had encountered during surgery?

Seth: No.

Grant: At any time you were there waiting did you hear any overhead pages concerning your wife?

Seth: I heard two prior to the phone call in the waiting room. The overhead page stated that a vascular surgeon was needed to the Operating Room four, stat.

Grant: Did you know Operating Room four was the operating room for your wife?

Seth: No, I didn't. A second overhead page came about five minutes after the first and I remember thinking that it was a long time between the two overhead pages, never realizing it could have been for Amy's procedure.

Grant: What was the second page for?

Seth: "We need a vascular surgeon to Operating Room four, stat; any vascular surgeon to Operating Room four, stat."

Grant: How much time elapsed between the two pages?

Seth: About five minutes.

Grant: Do you know who was making the overhead page?

Seth: I don't.

Grant: Had you received a call from the nurse before the overhead pages?

Seth: It was just seconds after the second overhead page.

Grant: And what you recall from that conversation was this female telling you there's been a complication (with Amy's) surgery and that Dr. Keel would be up to speak with you about it?

Seth: Yes.

Grant: Any other information other than that?

Seth: No. And I didn't inquire any other information. Call me naïve or whatever, but I didn't ask any further questions. I didn't even associate the overhead pages with my wife at that point.

Grant: What was the next information that you received about your wife's surgery?

Seth: It was a few minutes after the phone call into the waiting room. Two nurses or hospital staff members – dressed in scrubs – came up to me.

Grant: What did they say?

Seth: They sat down and told me that they were sent up to tell me that there was a slight complication with Amy's procedure and Dr. Keel would be up to speak with me shortly. I asked them if Dr. Keel was able to remove the septum, and one of them admitted that they weren't in the room with Amy, which I thought was odd because they were just basically giving me the same information I had received over the phone. But even at this point there was no indication that things were as bad as they were. Before they left, they assured me that things were under control and that Dr. Keel would be up to talk to me.

Grant: And these two nurses that came up, you said one of them you know was not involved with your wife's surgery. Do you know if the second nurse was involved with the surgery?

Seth: Neither.

Grant: Did you understand at that point that Dr. Keel was still in the operating room?

Seth: Yes.

Grant: So, you understood why she wasn't there with the two nurses?

Seth: Yes.

Grant: Are you still there by yourself at PMC?

Seth: Yes.

Grant: When is the next occasion you learn about Amy's surgery?

Seth: When Dr. Keel eventually made it up to see me.

Grant: How long was it before Dr. Keel came up to see you?

Seth: About 40 minutes to an hour.

Grant: Between the two nurses coming to see you and Dr. Keel?

Seth: The first time I saw Dr. Keel was after they (the nurses) departed.

Grant: Had you received any other information about your wife's condition before Dr. Keel arrived?

Seth: No.

Grant: So, you were still there at the hospital by yourself?

Seth: Yes.

Grant: Where do you and Dr. Keel have a conversation?

Steve: Object to the form.

Seth: It was in the surgery waiting room where I had been.

Grant: Was there anyone else present?

Seth: No.

Grant: Tell me what you recall.

Seth: Dr. Keel pretty much rehashed what the nurses already told me. The only other thing that she added was the procedure was no longer outpatient; that Amy was going to be staying in the hospital. And she told me they had to cut her abdomen open to do repairs and that Amy received a blood transfusion.

Grant: Anything else?

Seth: She said that Amy was in pretty good hands and that she had good doctors working on her. And before (Dr. Keel) departed she said that she was going to notify me before transporting Amy to the recovery room.

Grant: Was it your understanding that your wife was still in surgery at the time you were having this conversation with Dr. Keel?

Seth: Yes.

Grant: Dr. Keel tells you that there had been a complication during surgery?

Seth: Yes.

Grant: Did she explain to you what sort of complication had occurred?

Seth: That she saw blood and that a trocar malfunction was suspect to why she saw the blood in Amy's abdomen.

Grant: What was Dr. Keel's demeanor during your conversation with her that day?

Seth: It was still pretty much the same. There was nothing about her demeanor that gave me any concern.

Grant: Nothing about her demeanor you found to be inappropriate?

Seth: No.

Grant: In fact, would you say that that was your assessment of all your encounters with Dr. Keel?

Seth: Up to that point, yes.

Grant: Are there any future encounters that changed your mind about her demeanor?

Seth: My next encounter.

Grant: Dr. Keel tells you during this first conversation following surgery that your wife would have to stay in the hospital?

Seth: Yes.

Grant: Did she tell you how long?

Seth: No.

Grant: Dr. Keel tells you that your wife had required some blood transfusions during the surgery?

Seth: Yes.

Grant: Did she tell you how many?

Seth: No.

Grant: Dr. Keel tells you that your wife's in good hands and there are good doctors working on her; is that right?

Seth: Yes.

Grant: Did you understand who was working on her, what type of physicians were working on her at that time?

Seth: No.

Grant: Dr. Keel, when she left, did she tell you she was returning to the operating room?

Seth: As I understood it, because she was going to notify me when they moved Amy to recovery.

Grant: How long was that first conversation you had with Dr. Keel?

Seth: No longer than five minutes.

Grant: When was the next time you received any information about your wife?

Seth: When I returned to the hospital.

Grant: Did you at some point leave the hospital?

Seth: Yes.

Grant: At what point in time did you leave?

Seth: I received a call in the waiting room that told me Amy was still in surgery and that if I had not eaten lunch, then that was a good time to go. And I didn't have any cash with me, but we lived close by, so I went home to get lunch.

Grant: So, after your conversation with Dr. Keel, you received another phone call?

Seth: Yes.

Grant: Do you know who you were speaking with during that conversation?

Seth: No, I do not.

Grant: So, Amy was still in surgery at this time?

Seth: That was my understanding.

Grant: Had you called the surgical suite, or had you made any inquiry there of anyone at the hospital about her status before you received that phone call?

Seth: No, I hadn't.

Grant: So, you were just sitting there in the waiting room and you received another phone call?

Seth: Exactly. I was sitting there waiting to be notified when she was moved to recovery.

Grant: And someone just calls and tells you that she's still in surgery, that you can go grab lunch if you wanted to?

Seth: Right. It was the reason they called.

Grant: Did you ask them if you could leave the hospital and grab lunch, or did they just volunteer that?

Seth: Neither. I've already answered why I left.

Grant: So, you at that point leave the hospital, return to your home?

Seth: Yes.

Grant: Have lunch and come back to the hospital?

Seth: Yes. Well, I didn't have lunch, but I did return to the hospital.

Grant: You did go home?

Seth: Yes.

Grant: What did you do at home if you didn't have lunch?

Seth: Started to have lunch before I received another phone call at home.

Grant: And was the phone call from the hospital?

Seth: The phone call was from Dr. Keel's office. I was told to return to the hospital.

Grant: Did they give you any other information?

Seth: No.

Grant: How long had you been at home before you received the call from Dr. Keel's office?

Seth: Not more than ten minutes.

Grant: They just asked if this is Seth Larren, you tell them yes, and they said you need to return to the hospital?

Seth: Exactly.

Grant: No more information?

Seth: No.

Grant: No more discussion?

Seth: The person that I was speaking to identified herself as a nurse from Dr. Keel's office; I asked the person on the phone if everything was okay, and she told me she didn't have any information, except that they needed me to return to the hospital.

Grant: When you left the hospital, were there any other family members there at that time?

Seth: No.

Grant: When you returned to the hospital, were there any family members there other than yourself?

Seth: No.

Grant: After you return, who do you first speak with about your wife's condition?

Seth: Dr. Keel.

Grant: And what are you told?

Seth: That Amy had to be rushed back into surgery.

Grant: Did she tell you why?

Seth: Yes.

Grant: What did she say?

Seth: That they had completed operating on Amy, and that they had to give her a transfusion, that her blood pressure dropped, and this was why they rushed her back into surgery.

Grant: Was your wife still in surgery at the time you're having this conversation with Dr. Keel?

Seth: Yes. I understood that she had come out of surgery, gone to recovery, and had gone back into surgery and was in surgery as I was talking with Dr. Keel.

Grant: Did Dr. Keel explain to you why your wife's blood pressure had dropped and that it became necessary to take her back into surgery?

Seth: She made an effort to describe it, but I can't say I understood it at that time – because it hit me that Amy was in far worse shape than they had let on, or than

I had been led to believe. But I knew something was terribly wrong because the doctor's demeanor had changed.

Grant: What about Dr. Keel's demeanor had changed?

Seth: When I arrived back at the hospital I encountered her on my way to the elevators from the parking lot, and she saw me in the corridor and ran towards me. And she was trying to keep her panic under control, but it was here that I realized the worst.

Grant: Okay, so when you're there at the elevator you see Dr. Keel?

Seth: As I'm going towards the elevator.

Grant: And she's standing at the elevator?

Seth: No. I don't know where she was coming from. She was on the ground floor, perhaps trying to find me, but she saw me and came running towards me.

Grant: You said Dr. Keel was in a controlled, but panicked state?

Seth: Right. I could tell that something was wrong.

Grant: Urgency in her voice?

Seth: Yes.

Grant: Did Dr. Keel tell you how long she had been looking for you?

Seth: No, she didn't.

Grant: I guess if she had been searching through the hospital for you that could certainly have caused urgency in her voice that day, right?

Steve: Object to the form.

Seth: Possibly.

Grant: And in fact, she told you that she had been looking for you throughout the hospital?

Seth: She didn't say she was looking for me throughout the hospital, only that she had been trying to find me.

Grant: Any other information you learned from Dr. Keel during that encounter, other than (Amy's) blood pressure dropping and them taking her back into surgery?

Seth: No, and I resisted asking because I wanted full attention upon Amy.

Grant: Did Dr. Keel tell you which physicians were treating your wife at that time?

Seth: No.

Grant: Was it your understanding that Dr. Keel would be returning to surgery with Amy?

Seth: Based on (Dr. Keel's) next question of asking me where I was going to be, I presumed that she was going back to where Amy was. I told her that I was going to be in the waiting room and I wasn't going anywhere, and I wanted to be kept informed of everything from this point forward.

Grant: When's the next time you learn of any information about your wife's condition?

Seth: The next time was – some minutes after I returned to the waiting room the hospital administrator had come to greet me, but I didn't learn anything from her.

Grant: And who was the hospital administrator that met you?

Seth: I don't remember the woman's name.

Grant: She introduced herself as being the administrator for the hospital?

Seth: Yes.

Grant: What did she say to you?

Seth: She found me and introduced herself, and apologized for what was happening
           with Amy. I don't remember the specific conversation, but she provided me no
           new information as to what was going on with Amy; she asked me if I wanted
           to see a chaplain.

Grant: You say she apologized for what was happening. What did she say about that?

Seth: I believe she understood that Amy had come in for an outpatient surgery. She
           said something to the effect, "I'm sorry all of this is happening to you."

Grant: And the administrator didn't tell you any additional information regarding your
           wife's condition?

Seth: No. And I believe I asked her, but I got no new information.

Grant: At any time did the administrator place any blame or fault anyone for what was
           occurring with your wife?

Seth: No. But how likely is that?

Grant: Did the administrator, like Dr. Keel, tell you they were looking for you there in
           the hospital?

Seth: No.

Grant: Had you contacted any family members up to that point?

Seth: I called Amy's mother.

Grant: Anyone else?

Seth: No.

Grant: And when did you first call Amy's mother?

Seth: After my conversation with Dr. Keel in the corridor. Her mother was aware of the surgery and called me at home right after I received a call from Dr. Keel's office, because apparently, they called my mother-in-law at her residence looking for me before they reached me at home.

Grant: Did you speak with your mother-in-law when you were at home?

Seth: Yes, it was right after I hung up the phone with Dr. Keel's office, and before I even made it to the door to return to the hospital, the phone rang again, and it was my mother-in-law telling me the hospital is trying to find me and she was concerned why I was not at the hospital. I told her I was informed by a hospital staff member to go have lunch while Amy was still in surgery and told her I was on my way back to the hospital, and she wanted me to call her back as soon as I found out what was going on.

Grant: And that was the extent of the conversation?

Seth: Yes.

Grant: Do you have a second conversation with Amy's mother after your encounter with Dr. Keel?

Seth: Yes.

Grant: And does Amy's mother arrive at the hospital?

Seth: Yes.

Grant: What point in time did she arrive that day?

Seth: Perhaps mid to late-afternoon.

Grant: How long after your conversation with Dr. Keel?

Seth: About 45 minutes to an hour.

Grant: I take it you passed along what Dr. Keel had told you?

Seth: Yes.

Grant: Is Amy's mother there by herself or was Amy's father present also?

Seth: She was there by herself.

Grant: Had you received any more information about your wife's condition before Amy's mother arrived?

Seth: No.

Grant: When is the next time you receive information about your wife's condition.

Seth: When Dr. Keel comes into the waiting room – which, by this time, we were moved to a private waiting room.

Grant: And it's just you and your mother-in-law?

Seth: And a couple of Amy's friends.

Grant: Who called Amy's friends?

Seth: I believe my mother-in-law did.

Grant: Do you recall what friends are present?

Seth: Karyn Smith, and her sister, Karla.

Grant: And Amy's friends, do they accompany you and your mother-in-law to the private (waiting) room?

Seth: They arrived into the waiting room before anyone else had, including my mother-in-law.

Grant: So, they are present when Dr. Keel is talking with you about Amy's condition?

Seth: Yes.

Grant: And tell me what Dr. Keel told you.

Seth: Well, at this point she wasn't talking so much to me as she was Amy's mom. But she just repeated what she told me initially about the complication in Amy's surgery.

Grant: What did she say about it?

Seth: It was pretty much verbatim what she had told me earlier. And I guess Amy's mother, being more intuitive than I, asked how this could happen and Dr. Keel explained the procedure again and talked about this device that she used to enter the abdominal wall having a plastic sheath, and the fact that it was possible that the sheath malfunctioned to cause the injury.

Grant: Anything else?

Seth: Nothing.

Grant: Was it your understanding that Amy was out of surgery at the time you were having that conversation with Dr. Keel?

Seth: At the time we're having this conversation, I don't know exactly what's going on. I believed Amy was still in surgery.

Grant: You mentioned that Dr. Keel was talking to Amy's mother and not you. Do you know why she was talking to Amy's mom and not yourself?

Seth: Well, by that time I had already met with the chaplain, and I wanted to find out if he knew anything, but he didn't have anything to add to the information I already had. By the time Dr. Keel arrived to talk with Amy's family, I was pretty distraught, so though I was in the room, it was Amy's mom who wanted the information.

Grant: And Dr. Keel tells her that she had encountered a complication during the surgery?

Seth: Yes.

Grant: And then she went on to explain how she performed the surgery?

Seth: Yes.

Grant: And she mentioned something about a plastic sheath being on the end of one of the instruments?

Seth: Yes.

Grant: And how that plastic sheath was supposed to protect – keep it from inflicting any injury when they went inside?

Seth: Right.

Grant: But there had been some injury on the inside, because of the instruments they used?

Seth: Yes.

Grant: And the surgery they were doing afterwards was correcting those injuries?

Seth: That's correct.

Grant: I don't know if you were able to get a sense of it, but what was Dr. Keel's demeanor at that point in time?

Seth: That's a good question.

Grant: And maybe you don't know because you weren't really focused on that.

Seth: At that point, I wasn't actively trying to perceive that. I don't know. It wasn't panicky like the time I saw her before. I'd probably say at this point it was more defensive. I don't know if it was because she had accepted the fact that Amy was injured, or because she was dealing with Amy's mother, or because of unknowable circumstances or whatever.

Grant: Was there any yelling going on between your mother-in-law and Dr. Keel?

Seth: Not at all; absolutely not.

Grant: What about between Amy's friends and Dr. Keel?

Seth: No.

Grant: Did they have any questions of Dr. Keel?

Seth: No. They pretty much realized it wasn't their place to ask questions and were there only to support the family.

Grant: Was Amy's mother or her friends keeping any notes?

Seth: No. Not that I'm aware of.

Grant: When was the next time you received any information about Amy?

Seth: When we were still in the waiting room and Dr. Ferris came in to speak with us.

Grant: What did Dr. Ferris tell you?

Seth: He gave us the facts: that they worked on Amy, that she lost a lot of blood, that she sustained a lot of damage and significant trauma, that at that point the prognosis wasn't really good or hopeful. They had concerns for organ failure, multiple organ failure, system failure, possible brain damage. He talked about how the first 24 hours are the most critical for the patient. And probably as cordially as he could, told us that Amy would be continuously monitored and whatever. But by the time he left, we didn't have any real expectation that she would pull through.

Grant: What role did Dr. Ferris play in Amy's treatment?

Seth: I don't know, but I'm sure the records will tell you.

Grant: Was Amy out of surgery at the time you're having this conversation with Dr. Ferris?

Seth: At the time we're having this conversation I don't even know that Amy is out of surgery. I was told, and I'm not sure by whom, that I was going to be allowed to see her when she got to the recovery room, but at this time no family member had seen Amy since they took her off to surgery.

Grant: Did Dr. Ferris tell you what additional surgery had been performed?

Seth: I don't remember if he did.

Grant: You said Dr. Ferris mentioned that Amy lost a lot of blood. Did he quantify that in any way?

Seth: No.

Grant: Do you have any other conversations with Dr. Keel that day?

Seth: No.

Grant: At any point after that day, do you have additional conversations with Dr. Keel?

Seth: Yes.

Grant: Tell me about those.

Seth: I may have spoke with her once or twice on the 8th. She conversed with the family, including Amy's father, in the ICU waiting room on the evening of the 8th. She appeared to be trying to get a sense of the family's thoughts and said that she was sorry but sometimes these things happen and that Amy is just a very thin girl – which I found pretty amazing because at no time in the past did the doctor ever mention that Amy had to be a certain weight in order to have this recommended procedure done.

Grant: You mentioned that Dr. Keel went out of town for a period of time. What physician was covering for her when she was out of town?

Seth: I guess it was her partner, Dr. Finch.

Grant: Had you returned to work on a part-time basis before Dr. Keel left town?

Seth: I don't believe so. No.

Grant: It was a day or two after Dr. Keel left to go out of town that you returned to work part-time?

Seth: It was after that, yes.

Grant: Getting back to the 7th, you mentioned Dr. Ferris came and spoke to the family, updated them about Amy's condition. Did you receive any other updates that day, on the 7th, from other physicians about Amy's condition?

Seth: Not from other physicians.

Grant: Your updates would come from nurses?

Seth: Yes. Amy was in the ICU so we were able to finally be with her.

Grant: Did you ever see Amy when she was in the recovery room?

Seth: Yes.

Grant: How long after your conversation with Dr. Ferris did you first see Amy in the recovery room.

Seth: About 20 to 30 minutes.

Grant: Had Chris Resar and his wife arrived at the hospital before you saw Amy in the recovery room?

Seth: No.

Grant: Did you ever see any family members, friends, others that were there on Amy's behalf, get into an argument with hospital staff or physicians?

Seth: No, and I don't recall any event like that ever happening.

Grant: Did anyone at any time ever tell you about statements made during Amy's surgery?

Seth: No.

Grant: On the 7th, when you see Amy in ICU, is she returned to surgery that day?

Seth: No. She does not go back into surgery on that day.

Grant: At any point in time is she returned to surgery?

Seth: On the 8th.

Grant: And what is your understanding of why she was taken back to surgery on the 8th?

Seth: Her condition didn't improve that first night.

Grant: Did you stay at the hospital that evening?

Seth: Yes, I did.

Grant: The entire time?

Seth: Stay at the hospital the entire time?

Grant: Yes.

Seth: No, I didn't stay at the hospital the entire time.

Grant: And where did you go?

Seth: Most of my time I was at the hospital. There was one evening where Amy's family insisted that I go home and spend the night there, but it was agreed between Amy's mother and I on the first night that (Amy) wouldn't be there by herself. So, whether it was going to be me staying there or her mother, or some other family member, somebody was going to be there with her.

Grant: That first night, do you remember her mother being there and you returning home?

Seth: No, I was there.

Grant: You were there the first night?

Seth: Absolutely. I was there most nights, as any responsible husband would be. There was only one evening throughout her entire stay in the hospital where I didn't sleep at the hospital.

Grant: Okay. How were you informed that Amy was being returned to surgery on the 8th?

Seth: I was informed by Dr. Milton.

Grant: What was your understanding of why they were (returning) her to surgery?

Seth: My understanding was that they needed to go back in to do some exploring to determine why she wasn't improving. Internal bleeding was suspected.

Grant: Had you spoken with Dr. Keel before Dr. Milton tells you that they are going to return Amy to surgery?

Seth: I don't remember. I may have, early that morning on the 8th, but I'm not sure what Dr. Keel's role was at that point. I do know that they wouldn't perform surgery on Amy without my authorization and my agreeing to sign an Advanced Consent form. But perhaps my conversation that may have taken place with Dr. Keel that morning was for her to coach my thinking on allowing Amy to have the fourth surgery.

Grant: What do you mean her involvement was to coach you?

Seth: Like I said, I'm not for certain that I did see her that morning, but if I did – and I may have – they were not going to be able to perform the surgery without my consent, and-

Grant: I see. So, she was there talking with you, you think, about the surgery Dr. Milton was going to perform?

Seth: If I indeed talked to her that morning-

Grant: Okay. And I take it you have a pretty good recall of what happened on the 7th, as far as conversations with Dr. Keel; right?

Seth: Yes.

Grant: Would it be fair to say that conversations you had with Dr. Keel after the 7th, they all kind of start to run together?

Seth: To some degree, yes; at that point the relationship we had with her before the surgery wasn't the same as after the surgery.

Grant: Did that change because of her attitude or your attitude?

Seth: I think there were a lot of dynamics going on other than attitudes, so I don't believe you could pin it on anybody's attitude.

Grant: What would you pin it on?

Seth: The events of what happened. You know, my wife was severely injured and was probably about to die, and the doctor arguably responsible for injuring her is the same one whom we've had some incidents with before in the past. That tends to change the relationship, don't you think?

Grant: Did you notice any change in Dr. Keel's attitude after March 7th?

Seth: When she tried to pin Amy's injury on the fact that Amy was too thin in that conversation she had with Amy's dad on the evening of the 8th, and you couple that with her prior explanation about the malfunctioning plastic sheath over the trocar, her explanations of the initial injury weren't consistent to us, or at least to me. This leads me to believe she was thinking defensively and trying to construct a strategy before any investigation took place. Other than that, nothing else stands out worth commenting on.

Grant: Dr. Milton - - is he the physician that operated on Amy on March 8th, or do you know?

Seth: Yes.

Grant: And I take it you have a discussion with him after his surgery?

Seth: Yes.

Grant: And just tell us about that conversation.

Seth: After the surgery he comes up to the ICU waiting room where I am and tells me that everything went okay, that he repaired another abdominal blood vessel, a perforation to her colon, an iliac artery tear, and that from what he sees, she's going to do much better.

Grant: Before Dr. Milton's surgery, had Amy regained consciousness?

Seth: No. Not that I'm aware of.

Grant: And you stayed with her the entire night of the 7th?

Seth: Yes.

Grant: Did Dr. Milton at any point in time tell you what caused these punctures to the blood vessel and the colon?

Seth: Yes.

Grant: What did he say?

Seth: He said that – when he started describing all the things he had repaired, (I asked him) how all these multiple injuries happened, because it sounded like he had a list of things to repair. He began to explain the repair of the abdominal blood vessel and said the initial injury was deeper than they had first recognized. When describing the colon injury, he explained how the colon lays over itself several times and the straight-shot injury went through all these folds, resulting in injury to several spots on the colon which had to be run and repaired.

Grant: Anything else?

Seth: When describing the injury penetrating deeper than initially thought, he held his fingers five to six inches apart.

Grant: Do you know who did the first repair surgery on your wife?

Seth: No, I do not.

Grant: You didn't understand that Dr. Milton did the first repair?

Seth: Okay, the first vascular repair, Dr. Milton. I understand that.

Grant: On the 7th, then he came back the next day on the 8th did a second repair surgery to Amy?

Seth: Right.

Grant: Did you ask Dr. Milton, "Well, you know, why didn't you see this when you were there the first time repairing things?"

Seth: No.

Grant: Did anyone in your family ask that question of Dr. Milton?

Seth: No.

Grant: Did Dr. Milton tell you at any point in time that during his first surgery he checked to see if there were any injuries deeper than what he saw?

Seth: No.

Grant: You do recall Dr. Milton telling you, after his surgery on the 8th, that the initial injuries were deeper than they thought?

Seth: Yes.

Grant: Did Dr. Milton continue caring for Amy after that surgery?

Seth: Yes.

Grant: Any other physicians you're aware of that cared for her after that surgery on the 8th?

Seth: Yes. Dr. Edwards, Dr. Wales to some degree, and I don't know of any others.

Grant: At any time were any of the physicians critical of Dr. Keel's care of Amy?

Seth: Not in front of me.

Grant: So, then you're not aware?

Seth: No.

Grant: At any time did you ask those physicians about Dr. Keel's care of Amy?

Seth: No.

Grant: Did you like Dr. Milton?

Seth: Did I like him? Yeah, I mean, there was no reason for me not to like him. He was trying to repair the damage done to my wife. I think he may have underestimated the depth of Amy's injuries – but he was okay, I guess.

Grant: He seemed polite and professional during your interactions?

Seth: During our interactions, yes. Although I felt he thought pretty highly of himself – but that's just a personal opinion.

Grant: Same question with regards to Dr. Edwards and Dr. Wales. They were both polite and professional during your interactions?

Seth: Yes.

Grant: And their care and treatment were successful, was it not?

Seth: Yes. It was.

Grant: In fact, they were able to avoid her going into organ failure?

Steve: Object to the form. If you can, answer that.

Seth: As far as I know.

Grant: Okay. You're not aware of her going into organ failure, are you?

Seth: No.

Grant: Likewise, you're not aware of her suffering any brain damage as a result of this?

Steve: Object to the form of the question.

Grant: When do you recall her gaining consciousness?

Seth: About three or four days after the 7th.

Grant: When Dr. Milton first approached you on March 8th, told you, "We're going to have to take your wife back to surgery to find out what is causing her condition," had the attorneys from this office arrived at the hospital?

Seth: No.

Grant: They arrived after Dr. Milton had completed the surgery?

Seth: No.

Grant: It was during?

Seth: It was during.

Grant: Was anyone from this office – attorney, staff, other members of this office – present during any conversations the physicians had with the family?

Seth: Not that I'm aware of.

Grant: Were you given a list of questions to ask the physicians?

Seth: No.

Grant: Was anyone instructed to take notes while the physicians were talking to the family?

Seth: I do not know.

Grant: I think I may have asked you this before, but did you tell any of the physicians that were caring for your wife that you had contacted attorneys?

Seth: No.

Grant: Were you aware that the attorneys from this office sent a letter to Dr. Keel, in the hospital, on March 14th, while your wife was still at PMC?

Seth: No.

Grant: So, it was three or four days after surgery on the 8th that Amy first regained consciousness; right?

Seth: Yes.

Grant: And Amy told us this morning that in addition to being in a lot of pain, her left leg was painful to her?

Seth: She complained about a lot of things, but yes.

Grant: You remember her mentioning pain in her left leg?

Seth: Yes.

Grant: Did you ever discuss that condition with any of the physicians (or) nurses that were treating her there at the hospital?

Seth: Dr. Edwards.

Grant: What did Dr. Edwards tell you?

Seth: He didn't want to address it – or try to address it.

Grant: Did you or someone in the family or maybe even Amy mention to the nurses or the physicians there that she had previously injured her left knee?

Seth: I commented – and this was days later with Amy out of the ICU – it was baffling to me why she was having problems with that particular leg and why it was so swollen. I remember commenting aloud that she had injured her leg before but never had any problems with it. This injury I was referring to was the injury you repeatedly asked her about, the strain that she injured on the job, and this injury happened many months before Amy and I were married in July of 20xx. I didn't understand why it was an issue at this point in time since the hospital didn't find – or said they didn't find anything on the x-rays of her knee.

Grant: You remember mentioning to someone – hospital staff or a physician – that?

Seth: I remember thinking out loud. Someone overheard me, but I wasn't telling this to anyone specifically.

Grant: If it's recorded somewhere in Amy's medical records that she had sustained a previous injury to that left knee, they probably would have learned that from either talking with you or Amy. Fair enough?

Seth: Amy wasn't in a talkative mood. I was the one who commented about the prior injury, mind you, the injury was never a problem for her to the degree that the recent injury was.

Grant: Okay. When Amy was discharged home, was she sent home with a knee brace, a walker, a cane, anything of that nature?

Seth: A walker, at my request.

Grant: Was she able to walk at the time she left the hospital?

Seth: Not without assistance.

Grant: Assistance being the walker?

Seth: The walker or somebody helping her with support. She was not putting any of her weight on that leg. She was dragging it behind.

Grant: Had the physical therapist come into Amy's room to work with her before her release from the hospital?

Seth: Yes.

Grant: And as I understand it from Amy's testimony, she never returned to see Dr. Keel after her release from Presbyterian Hospital?

Seth: That's correct.

Grant: Do you recall who she saw, as far as an obstetrician-gynecologist, after her release from Presbyterian Hospital?

Seth: Dr. Porter, as a referral from our family doctor.

Grant: I think you told me earlier you went with your wife to see Dr. Porter, but you stayed in the lobby while she went back to see him?

Seth: Right.

Grant: Has she told you what occurred during that visit with Dr. Porter?

Seth: I inquired, and she said that she didn't care for him because he – she didn't think he was a good doctor; his tone, his attitude, bedside manner, and something he said to the effect that injuries like hers are known risks of a laparoscopic surgery. How could he say that without knowing all the details? It appears that the guy made up his mind before he had any details, and it doesn't surprise me that he's their so-called expert witness.

Grant: Why was she seeing Dr. Porter?

Seth: Like I said, she got the referral to follow up with a gynecologist. We were supposed to follow up with Dr. Keel, but Amy did not want to see her again and understandably so.

Grant: Any other obstetricians-gynecologists treated Amy after that, other than Dr. Reysa?

Seth: No.

Grant: We read a list of physicians during your wife's deposition, that she's treated with since her discharge from PMC. Do you recall any other physicians she's treated with that were not on that list?

Seth: I don't remember the list you read to her.

Grant: All right. Dr. Hanson, Dr. Anderson, Dr. Olsen, Dr. Porter, Dr. Dyer, Dr. Brock, Dr. Elliott, Dr. Bennett, Dr. Reysa., Dr. Sanders, Dr. Talbot.

Seth: Dr. Penner.

Grant: Your wife has been to the emergency room a couple of times?

Seth: A few, yes.

Grant: And those emergency room visits I think were at Lakeside North Hospital?

Seth: Yes.

Grant: Did you ever have occasion to return to University Hospital for emergency room treatment?

Seth: Yes.

Grant: Did you receive treatment at University?

Seth: We returned to University Hospital once, and we left before she got treated.

Grant: Tired of waiting in the ER?

Seth: Yes, but Amy's incision wounds prevented her from sitting upright, and she couldn't recline in those chairs the way they were designed. After nearly an hour of waiting, Amy couldn't take it anymore. So, the pain that forced us to go there ended up forcing us to leave because we couldn't get prompt treatment.

Grant: And it looked like to me, from reviewing the records, you went from University over to Lakeside North the same day?

Seth: Not the same day.

Grant: What caused your wife to go to University Hospital?

Seth: She was having persistent, ongoing pain in her leg.

Grant: Had she been to treat with any other physicians before going to University emergency room?

Seth: No, not for that.

Grant: You hadn't yet located a referral from Dr. Sanders for an obstetrician-gynecologist?

Seth: No. At that point we hadn't even seen Dr. Sanders yet.

Grant: Was your wife ever given a knee brace to wear on her leg?

Seth: From her emergency room visit at Lakeside North; yes.

Grant: And she was given instructions on how to wear that, was she not?

Seth: Yes, she was.

Grant: And I think she was told to wear that every day?

Seth: Yes, she was.

Grant: And did she wear it every day?

Seth: No. The pain was such that she couldn't stand anything touching her leg; not pants, not a sheet, and certainly not a brace, because in case you didn't know, she had nerve damage that affected the entire leg.

Grant: Who all has she treated with for her complaints of left leg pain?

Seth: Initially, Dr. Sanders, who continued treating her and referred us to Dr. Olsen and Dr. Hanson. She got a referral from Dr. Hanson to see Dr. Talbot, but he continued treating her. And from Dr. Olsen, she got a referral to Dr. Anderson and therapy instructions at the McConnell Rehabilitation Center, and he continued to treat her as well.

Grant: And the last time your wife received rehab treatment would have been when?

Seth: Sometime in 20xx.

Grant: Did any of the physicians you mention ever tell you what was causing your wife to have pain in her leg?

Seth: They had theories.

Grant: What were their theories?

Seth: That she had nerve damage in the left side of her pelvis, (the femoral nerve) that contributed to the ongoing pain in her leg.

Grant: Did they have a theory on what caused this nerve damage in the pelvic area?

Seth: No. If they did, they didn't voice it to us.

Grant: You may not be aware of this, but I'll just ask anyway. Did your wife at any time have a catheter placed on the inside of her left leg?

Seth: Yes. I had to sign a Consent form to authorize them to do that.

Grant: Were there any problems with that catheter in her left groin area that you were aware of?

Seth: Not at the time she was in the hospital.

Grant: Were you aware of any problems with that catheter after she was discharged from the hospital?

Seth: Yes.

Grant: What do you know about that?

Seth: Only that the placement of the catheter in the site on the left side of her pelvic area didn't make it into the artery or the vein or whatever it was they were trying to get it into, and then they ultimately had to go into the one on the right side.

Grant: And wasn't it also part of the theories from the physicians treating your wife for the left leg pain that this catheter they attempted to place in her left groin area could have caused this nerve damage which then led to your wife's complaints of pain?

Seth: It is possible.

Grant: That was one of the theories they talked about?

Seth: Yes.

Grant: Do you know if Dr. Milton's surgery that he did on March 7th, March 8th, do you know if that surgery caused this nerve damage in your wife's pelvic area?

Seth: No, I do not.

Grant: We talked with your wife this morning about her right eyelid drooping a little bit. Has any physician ever attributed her right eyelid droop to what occurred there in the hospital in March 20xx?

Seth: Not specifically, but the fact remains that the eye wasn't like that before the hospitalization of 20xx, but is afterwards.

Grant: Have you or your wife ever received an explanation for what causes that?

Seth: No. I do know that Dr. Hanson recognized it when he first saw Amy and he was very concerned by it; not only the drooping lid, but the frozen state of the eye – that is, the pupil not changing size with increased or decreased amounts of light.

Grant: But did he have a cause for that?

Seth: None that he shared with us.

Grant: Do you recall when she first developed this droopy right eyelid?

Seth: It wasn't noticeable until she first became conscious and began to open her eyes, days after her admittance into the hospital.

Grant: You said earlier that you had made some computer entries when drafting these answers to interrogatories. And one of the interrogatories we ask is for you to identify all health care personnel whom you feel have the opinion that the defendant properly managed Amy Larren's medical care, and your answer to that, "To the extent health care personnel have offered opinions regarding the defendant's care and treatment of Amy, Dr. Milton and Porter may feel that the defendant's care was acceptable." Why did you provide that answer?

Seth: Well, I felt that Dr. Milton, during our stay there at the hospital and even at Amy's follow-up visit with him, he seemed to be pressing us to go back to see Dr. Keel, and there was no reason for him to be doing so, in light of everything that happened. I felt he was leaning us towards going back to see her, even though it was clearly not our intention to do so.

Grant: Why was that statement made with regard to Dr. Porter?

Seth: Porter is obviously a doctor's doctor, and it's not likely that he'll ever admit to a situation where he thinks the treating physician is at fault. Amy's injuries were undeniably terrible, and yet this doctor's cavalier attitude about her scars and the depth of her injuries was very robotic. Those comments he made to Amy (during her examination appointment) was an obvious reason we would feel this way, but I've never met Dr. Porter and me and my wife never discussed anything about him other than that moment when we first left his office.

Grant: From your conversations with Dr. Milton, he told you the same thing Dr. Keel did with respect to these injuries, that they were a complication of her procedure, correct?

Steve: Object to the form.

Grant: Before your first phone call with Chris Resar, is it fair to say that the only information you had about your wife's medical condition, you had learned from conversations with Dr. Keel?

Seth: Yes.

Grant: The pharmacies that we went over with your wife, the one at Wal-Mart and the one at Walgreen's, are you aware of any other pharmacies that you guys have utilized to fill her prescriptions?

Seth: I thought about that, and I don't believe there are any others. There is more than one Walgreen's location where we had prescriptions filled, but I believe their computer systems are networked together.

Grant: Have you ever been involved in any previous litigation? Have you ever sued anyone before?

Seth: No.

Grant: Has anyone ever sued you?

Seth: Yes.

Grant: What was the nature of that lawsuit, as you understand it?

Seth: I was in a vehicular wreck during an ice storm in _ _ _ County back in 20xx. No one was hurt, but I admitted to not allowing my windows enough time defrost. The case never made it to court.

Grant: Is that the only time you've been sued?

Seth: Yes, as far as I know.

Grant: Any workers' compensation claims?

Seth: No workers' compensation claims.

Grant: Ever been charged or convicted of a crime?

Steve: Object to the form.

Seth: Never.

Grant: I'm going to pass the witness.

Direct Examination begins by defense counsel, Ms. S. Short, representing Northwest Presbyterian Hospital. Here are some of the questions asked by Ms. Short during this deposition. These questions do not include every single question asked by Ms. Short, but it provides a basic insight into the defense of PMC. Because of space limitations, I will not record any of my responses.

Short: *You mentioned that your wife had seen a Dr. Penner?*

          As I understand it, he prescribed her some medication?

          You told us earlier this afternoon about how you and your wife presented to the hospital and some of the events that transpired prior to your wife going into surgery there at Presbyterian Hospital. Are you critical of anything that the preoperative hospital staff, nursing staff, did or didn't do for your wife?

Have any physicians that have seen your wife been critical of anything that the operating room staff did or didn't do for your wife?

Have you learned from any source – in other words, have you heard that a critical statement with respect to the OR staff was made to another family member?

Now, with respect to the recovery room staff, as I understand it you were in fact allowed to go back and visit your wife while she was in the recovery room; true?

During that visit, can you describe for me how your wife looked and what was going on?

Did she have blood infusing? In essence, did she have a blood transfusion hanging?

Do you remember having any discussion with any of the recovery room nurses that were in attendance during your visit?

Do you have any estimation as to how long you were in the recovery room?

Do you remember seeing any of your wife's physicians in the recovery room during your visit?

From your perspective, was there anything that the recovery room nurses did or didn't do for your wife that you were critical of?

From your perspective, was there anything that the ICU nursing staff did or didn't do for your wife that you are critical of?

Now there came a point in time when your wife was transferred out of the ICU into a regular hospital bed; true?

With respect to the nursing staff that cared for your wife after she was transferred out of the ICU, are you critical of anything that they did or didn't do for your wife?

What kind of complaints are you talking about? People not being fast enough or Johnny-on-the-spot?

Did she actually fall to the floor?

Did she hurt herself in any way?

I was going to ask you who washed her hair?

There was an entry in your wife's medical records, and I think it's dated the 15th of March, that says "Care coordinator called insurance company BC" – I'm assuming that means Blue Cross, and then there's an 1-800 number, "per husband's request... left message for return." Do you have any recollection as to why you would have someone from the hospital call the insurance company?

I asked your wife this question, and I apologize if you've been asked it already. Did you receive any phone calls from any bill collectors on behalf of any of the physicians or hospital treating your wife?

Do you feel like you or your wife have been hounded in any regard by bill collectors seeking payment for your wife's medical expenses?

Are you critical of anything that Dr. Milton did or didn't do?

Since your wife's hospitalization in March of 20xx, have you done anything to try and learn something more about Dr. Keel, such as any type of investigation?

I don't mean to misrepresent your wife's testimony, but it's my recollection that she made a comment to us earlier today that she's given some thought about returning to see Dr. Vickers, the psychologist? Has there been some discussion recently about her going back to see Dr. Vickers or someone else like Dr. Vickers?

Since the birth of your son, has she been a good mother?

Has she been able to take care of your son? I mean, her health problems aren't preventing her from taking care of your son?

Have you had an opportunity, Mr. Larren, to read the transcripts of the depositions taken of Dr. Milton and Dr. Lister?

Do you know how Dr. Wales came to be involved in your wife's care?

Do you have any sense with as to the number of physicians that showed up to take care of your wife simply because of the emergency situation?

I assume you're awfully appreciative that they did that?

Do you have any sense as to the numbers of units or volume of blood transfusions that your wife needed?

Can you tell me why you have sued Presbyterian Hospital?

With respect to the questions asked by Ms. Short, there seemed to be an effort to try and distance or separate the hospital's level of care from that of Dr. Keel's. From Mr. Grant's method of questioning, it appeared as if he was trying to deflect some of Amy's injuries away from Dr. Keel and onto Dr. Milton or other doctors. It's no secret how these doctors and other medical practitioners tend to lock arms when they smell a lawsuit on the horizon. It is surprising, however, that in rare situations, especially when the lawsuit advances as far as ours, like crabs they can become cannibalistic.

CHAPTER 25

Depositions: Dr. Keel & Dr. Porter

The depositions of Dr. Keel, the primary defendant, and Dr. Porter, the defense's expert witness, were taken in the early part of 20xx, roughly two years after Amy's botched surgery. Space constraints limit my ability to print the deposition responses of Dr. Keel and Dr. Porter in a detailed format as I have done with my own deposition and Amy's, so I will only summarize the substance of their testimonies. While I have not had the opportunity to view every deposition taken in our case, I have had to chance to read the depositions of Dr. Keel and Dr. Porter. The summary of their testimonies is based on information they provided in their depositions and also based on my discussion with my attorney who informed me of the impact these depositions may have on our case.

Both physicians, Dr. Keel and Dr. Porter, were prepared for the questioning by my attorney and knowledgeable of what it was they wanted to accomplish: that is, they didn't want to do us any favors by helping our attorneys in their depositions. But the facts of the case had to be pursued, and in spite of their big $10 words and their clinical expertise, the evidence of Amy's horrible injuries cannot be denied. There were answers to be had, in addition to the truth that needed to be revealed, and while we were not able to get an answer on how Amy's knee injury happened, other aspects of the case materialized to help our attorneys paint a picture of how to present this case to a jury to prove negligence.

Dr. Keel's deposition was taken many days before Dr. Porter's, after several attempts to pin down a date for her to provide her testimony. Her schedule kept conflicting with the dates of my attorney, Steve, who would be deposing her. He was very thorough, and unrelenting with Dr. Keel's uncooperativeness. Dr. Keel herself, in providing her deposition, was very evasive, defensive and at times even antagonistic. There were several times that our attorney, Steve, had the court reporter certify questions that her attorney, Mr. Grant, instructed her not to answer. The tone of the deposition, based on my reading of the transcript, was very confrontational. There was even one point where the doctor was becoming so uncooperative, that Steve demanded to go off the record. My guess is that he threatened to end the deposition and go directly to the judge. After about ten minutes the deposition was resumed, and the hostile tone seemed to taper off.

Many questions were asked of Dr. Keel during her deposition. Steve went deep into questioning of the doctor about the first D&C she performed on Amy in August of 20xx and the emergency D&C performed in December of 20xx, the same year. Dr. Keel was in a quandary to explain it without admitting fault because it was Dr. Keel herself who presented a second, optional explanation as to why the emergency D&C in December was necessary. The clinically accepted reason for the emergency D&C performed in December was offered by the ER physician at University Hospital, Dr. Bennett: Amy was in the process of miscarrying and the recent prior HSG procedure performed by Dr. Keel contributed to this miscarriage. The second explanation offered by Dr. Keel was her own failure to properly perform the first D&C back in August, although she didn't word it as I have here. In either case, her mistake forced the second D&C in December, suggesting some form of negligence even before the botched surgery in March, three months later.

Regarding the laparoscopic surgery on the morning of March 7th, Dr. Keel was asked to describe in detail the instrumentation and technique employed when performing this procedure and what happened next after it was determined that Amy was injured. The doctor described the procedure but resisted answering several direct questions relating to when she recognized something was wrong. It appeared that the doctor didn't know; whenever she finally realized there was a problem, she called for her partner to come assist her. In the discharge summary, the doctor reports that her partner was readily available, but her deposition proved that the doctor's partner arrived later than initially admitted and that the doctor failed to alert other, more readily available surgeons.

Dr. Keel was asked why she suspected a malfunctioning trocar was the reason for Amy's initial injury even though the doctor admitted she never encountered a malfunctioning trocar before. She was asked if she had saved the trocar since she suspected that it malfunctioned, but the doctor discarded the device. The doctor was also asked why, if she never encountered a malfunctioning trocar, she would determine that this was the cause to Amy's initial abdominal injury. Discovery had shown that the trocar used in Amy's procedure is covered by a protective spring-loaded plastic sheath. If it was going to malfunction it would have malfunctioned to *prevent* injury rather than cause it. Dr. Keel admitted that this reason was "only the best thing that she could come up without conducting her own discovery" as to why the injury occurred.

During Dr. Keel's questioning, she made remarks that were less professional than I would have expected. She seemed to make a very big deal of the fact that I had left the hospital for lunch and found it very "suspicious." She commented about Amy and I not being very "intuitive people" during our consultation visit and in general. She also claimed that when I arrived at her office to obtain copies of Amy's medical records, I had done so with lawyers accompanying me, which is not true. My attorney, Steve, actually caught her making up another excuse right there on the spot during the deposition and when he called her on it, she admitted her excuse was something she hadn't thought of before.

Continuing in his deposition of Dr. Keel, Steve inquired about the doctor having any prior malpractice complaints charged against her, her relationship with Dr. Porter and the typewritten portion of her office's medical records on Amy. Dr. Keel commented that a prior malpractice charge against her was from when she was a resident and she admitted to being Dr. Porter's protégé and he her professional mentor. When questioned about the typewritten portion of Amy's medical records from her office, Dr. Keel said this was done to record specifics of her consultation appointment with Amy and I; she asserted that even though it was different than the other consistent parts of the medical records it was not placed there in hindsight in efforts to "cover her bases."

Dr. Keel also claimed in her deposition testimony that she entered Amy's abdomen only once with the laparoscope. But our expert witness claims that there is absolutely no way that Amy's multiple internal injuries could have occurred with only one entry attempt. In fact, our expert was perplexed as to how Dr. Keel could claim a single entry when any practicing physician could conclude that Amy's injuries were caused by multiple entry efforts into her abdomen.

Here are the questions our attorney, Steve, had the court reporter to certify. These are the questions asked by our attorney of Dr. Keel at her deposition, which were not answered satisfactorily or sufficiently. These questions, since the answers provided were not sufficient, are the ones that will be probed further as the case and trial develop.

My question was if you disagreed with anything, as you sit here today, in reviewing that deposition right now, having reviewed it sometime today, is there something that you disagree with that Dr. Lister testified to or Dr. Milton testified to?

I'm asking you with respect to the medical records you reviewed, is there something that you can testify to right now, having reviewed them today, that you disagree with?

Can you answer for me today, other than the one example that you have given that Presbyterian likes to have the history and physical the day of the procedure, any other responsibilities that you have as a physician in completing medical records for patients you treat at Northwest Presbyterian Medical Center?

So, your comment about lots of people looked at the form and no one caught it, that's not based on any kind of fact that you have or knowledge that you have about the number of people that looked at the form; you're basically guessing that lots of people looked at the forms?

What discussion have you had with your husband about Amy's case?

Dr. Porter was deposed and had the opportunity to review Dr. Keel's deposition beforehand. Perhaps the most extraordinary thing out of his testimony was the fact that Dr. Porter said that Dr. Keel's treatment of Amy did not fall below any standard of care, even though she skipped a step that he always performs when doing this same laparoscopic procedure. Insufflating is the filling of gas into a bodily cavity for medical treatment purposes. How this would apply to the surgery Amy had on March 7th is by insufflating the abdomen, a separation occurs between the abdominal wall and inner organs. This space acts as a buffer so that the doctor performing the surgery can better determine, after entering the abdominal cavity, exactly where they are in terms of the positioning of the organs.

Dr. Porter admits that he always insufflates anytime he performs this procedure. He replied affirmatively that all the partners in his practice do so as well and that it is a requirement for every doctor within his practice. He even admitted that during Dr. Keel's training as a resident under him, all the residents were required to insufflate when performing a laparoscopic surgery. He had no idea or reason as to why Dr. Keel would deviate from this basic step in the procedure, yet he stands by his belief that she violated no care standard when giving Amy the laparoscopic surgery. It doesn't sound very coherent to me, but he's the one who'll have to explain this to a jury.

Further revelations in our case found that the hospital had not ordered blood for the surgery even though there was a known risk of blood loss for this type of procedure. Only when it was realized/determined that Amy needed a transfusion did the hospital staff attempt to get blood products into the operating room.

CHAPTER 26

Our Case Today

So, as it is today, our case has its foundation. As Amy gets better, the value of our case diminishes – according to our attorney. Nonetheless, through painstakingly slow discovery, the case has developed as follows:

1. Dr. Keel lost control of her tool during the surgery, for a procedure that was not likely needed, based on testimonial evidence collected from the defendant and additional subjects.

2. The doctor shows evidence of significant doubt about how the injury occurred and says that she kept mentally going over it. The doubt outweighs her confidence, which is contrary to a doctor who unmistakably knows they performed everything correctly in a procedure.

3. The doctor made an effort to blame it on a malfunctioning trocar, which would have actually *prevented* further injury rather than caused it had the device really malfunctioned.

4. Dr. Keel admitted she never experienced or saw a trocar that had malfunctioned and failed to save the one she claimed malfunctioned.

5. There is the question of why Dr. Keel didn't insufflate Amy's abdomen prior to driving the scope into the abdominal wall, even though insufflating is the technique that was taught while she trained as a resident under Dr. Porter.

6. Dr. Porter admits that he's always insufflated and has always taught this. All the doctors in his practice insufflate during this kind of procedure and he admits that he personally wouldn't do a laparoscopy without first insufflating.

7. Dr. Keel testified that she only went into the abdomen once, even though our expert witness claims that the depth and type of injuries Amy endured could not have occurred unless multiple entries were attempted.

8. Dr. Porter himself, the expert witness for Dr. Keel, says that he's never seen injuries consistent with Amy's during a laparoscopic procedure, even though he contends that no negligence occurred.

9. During her testimony, Dr. Keel made last-minute explanations that Amy's physiology is somehow different than common physiology for a woman similar to her age, weight, and height, even though Dr. Keel's notation under the *General Appearance* section of the *History & Physical Report* in Amy's medical record reads that Amy is a well-developed, thin, white female in no acute distress.

10. Dr. Keel admits that if Amy was not pregnant in November, then the first D&C she performed on Amy back in August was done so incompletely, making the emergency D&C in December a necessity.

There's other evidence that may be coming forth, but as it stands now, our attorneys seem confident with the evidence we currently have. Still, despite all the evidence we have in our favor, the defense promises to be formidable. These legal firms for which the attorneys work are the firms of choice for doctors in medical malpractice litigation. The doctors use these people for a reason and pay big dollars for representation. But our attorneys also argue that when these guys lose, they tend to lose big. This aside, I will repeat my earlier statement that there are no winners in a malpractice lawsuit.

CHAPTER 27

Final Thoughts

Despite what your beliefs might be about Dr. Keel, I don't want to portray her as an evil, mean-spirited individual. Surely, she isn't perfect, and her attitude changed negatively towards us after we filed suit, but prior to that she appeared to be everything we wanted in a doctor. She was kind and seemed to listen, even though the longer we allowed her to treat Amy the more her competence seemed to wane. I suspect she was overworked and had too many patients to treat from her practice. Still, the fact that we liked Dr. Keel probably caused us to overlook some disturbing signals that manifested earlier on in her medical assessment and treatment of Amy, such as her inability to diagnose a pregnancy in November of the year prior to Amy's botched surgery, and my conversation with her after the emergency D&C in December of the same year.

An argument that will no doubt arise from our malpractice case is the argument of whether Dr. Keel is a good physician or a poor one. When trial occurs, the defense will make efforts to put Dr. Keel in the best light possible. They will bring in former or current patients of Dr. Keel's to testify that she provided them exceptional service. This is fine; however, the question at hand is whether Dr. Keel was a good doctor for Amy. I believe the evidence speaks for itself.

There are some tough lessons we learned from this ordeal. With respect to the treating physician, here are some points we wish we heeded earlier in Amy's many office visits and clinical procedures:

Get referrals for medical specialists – If you can, get referrals from family, friends, or other people you trust when selecting a doctor, especially one as important as an OB/GYN. If family and acquaintances can vouch for the doctor based on their own experiences, then it's likely you will get the same level of care and competence.

Ask Questions – Ask questions of your doctor about any health issues related to you. Ask the doctor if he/she has ever been in a malpractice lawsuit. Trust your instincts if the doctor tends to be hesitant to answer a question or can't provide you a simple yes or no answer. Don't be afraid of offending your doctor if you ask him to explain something again and again, until you understand it sufficiently. His pride isn't worth the risk of your health or your life. If the doctor is offended by any legitimate question you ask, then it is an important indication to change doctors.

Get a second opinion – Always, always, always get a second opinion on a non-terminal health issue before agreeing to a procedure. It is worth the time, effort and extra cost, because if another doctor tells you something different than the first, it immediately lets you know that a discrepancy exists between two licensed professionals; you might need to get a third, fourth or fifth opinion before making a sound decision to go through with a procedure. Dr. Reysa, Amy's current OB/GYN, told us that as far as he was concerned, Amy could have a baby anytime she wanted to without any surgical intervention – and this was *after* her botched surgical event in March. Dr. Reysa successfully treated Amy's first successful pregnancy and is said to have delivered more babies in our state than any other physician. Furthermore, Dr. Reysa has *never* had a lawsuit filed against him. Imagine the pain and heartache Amy and I could have avoided if we only took the time to follow this advice of getting a second opinion.

Do your own research – For thorough understanding of recommended surgical procedures, perform your own research before your consultation appointment with your doctor. Not only is it worth the time, it is quite easy. WebMD.com is one of many good internet sources to find out more information about medical procedures physicians can perform on a person. It can also give you a basis for asking intelligent questions of the physician at the consultation appointment.

Be prepared – Know what to do beforehand if you suspect medical malpractice. This book contains good information and recommendations on what to do and how to be prepared if you – heaven forbid – become the victim of medical injury. No person that I have ever talked to in my entire life ever claims they want to be the victim of any doctor's negligence, and no doctor that I know of who is sane ever wants to be charged with malpractice, so it is likely that you may never be in this situation. But if you ever are, just know what to do. Part of knowing what to do is knowing exactly which attorney or law firm you will contact if you were injured, because promptness is an important asset for the plaintiff in a malpractice matter.

Hire a specialty law firm – If you ever become the victim of a medical injury case, hire a law firm that specializes in medical malpractice litigation. The attorneys I chose to hire were contacted for me in a very constrained period of time. They appear to be performing a decent job for us, but I question if I would have chosen them had I had the time to do my own research to find a legal team. Many of their clients are insurance companies, petroleum companies, banks and other corporate outfits, but they simply aren't well known for personal injury cases. Under the situation for which we found ourselves, I'm confident they will do a good job for Amy and me.

Resist making unsolicited records – Unless asked by your attorney, never try to help your attorney by collecting unsolicited written statements, recorded or the like. This information will have to be disclosed to the defense's legal team if you provide recorded information to your attorney. It is to your benefit for your legal team to keep certain aspects of the trial strategy confidential from the defense's legal team. If you must make personal notes, keep them private. Turning them over to your attorney can make them exhibits to the case. Unless requested by your counsel, destroy unsolicited records before you begin answering Interrogatories and Requests for Production by the defense counsel. The defense will ask you about these and demand for you to turn them over and you have a legal obligation to comply.

Do make videos – Videos help record evidence thereby supplementing your testimony of suffering. I failed to take any video of Amy in her many moments of suffering; and if I had, it would have spoken volumes more than anything I, Amy or our attorney could say about how terrible the injuries were for her. "Pain and suffering" is a cojoined term that tends to just roll off the tongue, similar to the lexicon of other pairs, such as "wind and rain" or "nuts and bolts." We all know what pain and suffering is, but it's used so often in malpractice cases that it tends to lose the true significance of its meaning. Nights when I'd arrive home from work and found Amy in the total dark, lying in our bed in a fetal position, crying profusely because of the pain that wasn't being controlled by the medication, or those many nights where she couldn't sleep because of the agonizing pain that kept her awake, cannot fully be captured by words; even photographs fall short of telling the entire story. There is no dispute that with a video, the display of agony cannot be contested or explained away by some slick, high-paid defense lawyer. The jury sees for itself the degree of real pain, real suffering and real mental anguish that exists because of the medical injury. Where the defense can try to make light of the situation, the video communicates what words cannot. As a result, the compassion and humanity of the jury should extend to the plaintiff, which may translate to a larger award.

Prayer and meditation – The reality of our human existence is that we are physical beings with a non-physical essence to our existence. Medical science has at least advanced to the point where this notion is less debatable today than it was even 30 years ago. So, it really does help to nurture the spirit when surviving through a medical injury. Prayer to God and meditation on His promises in scripture helps tremendously if you or a loved one is experiencing loss as a result of a medical malpractice injury. Arming yourself in prayer and meditation can greatly help you weather the storm of opposition you will receive when attempting to advance your case.

Finally, our story is both unique from any other malpractice case and in ways, like every malpractice case. It is unique to other malpractice cases in the sense of how it happened, how it has evolved, and how we have evolved because of it. It is similar to other malpractice cases in the sense of how the practitioners locked arms to protect each other, the untold pain and anguish, and the long, challenging road to recovery.

Amy and I can look back at many things from the time she first began seeing Dr. Keel. We thank God for His divine intervention in helping us get through the moments of pain, emotional anguish, bewilderment, anger, frustration and financial shortcomings that have befallen us because of what happened, not only in the hospital on March 7th, but incidents before and since then. We have overcome them all. Only with God's help and the people He put in our lives at the time were we able to do so.

Imagine going from a situation where your wife is about to die in the cold confines in a hospital room, to the extraordinary joy of her finally birthing into the world a new life some three years later! Amy successfully gave birth our first-born child – a little baby boy. Her painful pregnancy, marked by many hospital visits throughout, was considered high-risk due to the internal scarring suffered from the botched surgery in March. Almost exactly three years later, in March, our greatest blessing was realized. Little Seth Michael was born at University Hospital at 7:58 p.m. weighing in at 6 pounds, 10 ounces. He arrived despite a dire situation three years earlier that could very well have prevented his birth.

In January of the year that Little Seth Michael was born, my dad took sick and was diagnosed with lung cancer in February of that same year. Dad passed away only 5 days before Seth Michael was born, so he never got the chance to see his grandson. Dad anticipated the birth of his new grandson, but he also knew the reason for which he was hospitalized. While hospitalized, he apologized to me that he wasn't going to get the opportunity to see his grandson. I told Dad that he has nothing to apologize for and that as far as I was concerned Little Seth would know everything about him and I promised that I would take care of his grandson, as well as my mother. Like I prayed for Amy's recovery three years earlier, I prayed for my dad's recovery – but God had different plans. As Dad deteriorated over the course of 5 weeks from that diagnosis in January, my prayer became such that if it was my father's time to depart us, then please let it happen fast. Maybe this was also an answered prayer.

My dad missing the birth of his grandson *could* be the greatest tragedy of this entire ordeal. It is testimony to the high personal stakes that exist in a malpractice incident. The impact that a doctor's error can have on an individual's life extends far beyond what happens in the hospital or the setting where the injury occurred. Dad's departure naturally took a large piece of me when he passed away, but the birth of my son so soon after Dad's departure reminded me that even in a loss, God can bless us with a fresh start.

Today, when my son looks at the wedding pictures of Amy and I with my dad in them, he points to dad in the pictures and calls his name. "Dad!" he says, and I tell him that dad is in heaven with Jesus, and we will see him someday when we get there. My father was an extraordinary Christian man and based on the promises of Scripture, we know we will see him again. This is the hope that we Christians have for those Christians passing on before us. Dad was mindful of this promise as he took sick. This mountain of a man laid in a bed where he was stripped of all his physical strength. But while he was weak physically, he was at his strongest emotionally and spiritually. He died well, with the knowledge that he was going into the presence of a personal and loving God, who loves us enough to have sent His only begotten son to die in our place as a sacrifice from the eternal judgment of our sin. And it might not be politically correct to say so, but this is an assurance that *only Christians* have.

Because our malpractice case has yet to advance to court or mediation, the conclusion of our story is yet to be finalized. Depending on how well this book is received, I am prepared to write a follow-up/conclusion of our story, where I will include the detailed depositions of Dr. Keel and Dr. Porter. This second book will be titled, *Botched II: Terrible Malpractice Injury Cases and a Survivor's Story Conclusion*. By the time this first book is published, we will be on the threshold of having our case resolved. How will our case turn out? Time will tell. Yet, regardless of whether we are awarded millions, nothing, or something in between, nobody can ever truly call us winners. We are only survivors, fortunate enough to have been blessed with a second chance. And notably, a second chance to build a life with my wife, whom I love very much, and the beautiful child she gave me, is truly worth many times more than any amount of compensation we could ever receive from a malpractice case.

GLOSSARY

Actual Damages

Compensation for losses that can readily be proven to have occurred and for which the injured party has the right to be compensated.

Attorney

A person legally appointed by another to act as his or her agent in the transaction of business, specifically one qualified and licensed to act for plaintiffs and defendants in legal proceedings.

Botch

To ruin through clumsiness or to make or perform clumsily, bungle. To repair or mend clumsily. To blunder, mess up or ruin awkwardly.

Botched

Past-tense form of 'botch'.

Cannula

A flexible tube, usually containing a trocar at one end that is inserted into a bodily cavity, duct, or vessel to drain fluid or administer a substance such as a medication.

Central Line

A catheter (tube) that is passed through a vein to end up in the thoracic (chest) portion of the vena cava or in the right atrium of the heart. The possible complications of a central venous line include air in the chest (pneumothorax) to a punctured lung, bleeding in the chest (hemothorax), fluid in the chest (hydrothorax), bleeding into or under the skin (hematoma) and infection. If the line becomes disconnected, air may enter the blood and cause problems with breathing or a stroke. A central venous line is also called a central venous catheter, though sometimes, the "venous" is omitted and it is called a central line or central catheter.

Compensatory Damages

See *Actual damages*.

Consent for Medical Treatment Form

A form requiring the signature of a patient party that establishes consent to a surgical or medical procedure after achieving an understanding of the relevant medical facts and the risks involved.

Contingency

The condition of being dependent on chance or uncertainty. In a legal sense, lawyers who work on a contingency basis forfeit payment for legal services until the subject case is won in court or a settlement offer is reached. The attorney is paid a percentage of the monies won or settled from the case.

Court Reporter

A stenographer who makes a verbatim record and transcription of proceedings, as in a court.

Damage

Physical harm caused to something in such a way as to impair its value, usefulness, or normal function.

Damages

Money ordered to be paid as compensation for injury or loss. Also, the demonstrative loss or harm that has a quantifiable value such that a monetary payment can be made.

Defendant

A person or institution against who an action is brought in a court of law; the person being sued or accused.

Defensive Medicine

Diagnostic or therapeutic measures conducted primarily as a safeguard against possible malpractice liability; the practice of ordering medical tests, procedures, or consultations of doubtful clinical value in order to protect the prescribing physician from malpractice suits.

Deposition

Testimony under oath, especially a statement by a witness that is written down or recorded for use in court at a later date.

Dereliction of Duty

Whenever doctors fail to maintain the agreed-upon relationship with a patient or overstep their boundaries.

Direct Causation

The process of determining whether a physician's actions were the direct result of harm towards the patient.

Disability

A disadvantage or deficiency, especially a physical or mental impairment that prevents or restricts normal achievement.

Discovery

The compulsory disclosure of pertinent facts or documents to the opposing party in a civil action, usually before a trial begins; the methods used by parties to a civil or criminal action to obtain information held by the other party that is relevant to the action.

Discovery Request

– See *request for production*.

Disfigure

To mar or spoil the appearance or shape of; the act of damaging the appearance or surface of something; a common result of a botched surgery, often an awardable offense.

Doctor

– See *physician*.

Duty of Care

A doctor's duty to care for their patient, requiring adherence to a standard of reasonable care while performing any acts that could foreseeably harm others.

Electromyogram (EMG)

A test measuring the electrical impulses of muscles at rest and during contraction. Nerve conduction studies, which measure nerve conduction velocity, determine how well individual nerves can transmit electrical signals.

Exhibits

Production evidence for a case

Extremis (In Extremis)

A medical term meaning, at the point of death.

Faith

Confident belief in the truth, value, or trustworthiness of a person, idea, or thing; Christian Theology: the trust in God and in His promises as made through Christ and the Scriptures by which humans are justified or saved.

Femoral nerve

A nerve that supplies sensation to the outer portion of the thigh.

Fracture

A medical condition in which there is a partial or complete break in the continuity of any bone in the body, most often happening when more force is applied to the bone than the bone can take, typically caused by falls, trauma, or the result of a direct blow to the body.

Gynecologist

– See OB/GYN.

Gynecology

The area of medicine that involves the treatment of women's diseases, especially those of the reproductive organs. It is often paired with the field of obstetrics, forming the combined area of obstetrics and gynecology.

Hemothorax

Accumulation of blood in the pleural cavity (the space between the lungs and the walls of the chest).

Hippocratic Oath

An oath embodying the duties and obligations of physicians, usually taken by those about to enter upon the practice of medicine; an oath of ethical professional behavior sworn by new physicians and attributed to Hippocrates.

Hypotension

Abnormally or severely low arterial blood pressure.

Hysterosalpingogram (HSG)

A diagnostic x-ray procedure performed to determine whether the fallopian tubes are open and to see if the shape of the uterus is normal. The test includes a filling of the uterus with liquid containing iodine for contrast. It is usually done after menses have ended, but before ovulation, to prevent interference with an early pregnancy.

Hysteroscopy

A procedure to see inside the uterus (the womb) using a viewing tube that is inserted into the vagina up through the cervix into the uterus.

Iliac (femoral) artery

A large artery that starts in the lower abdomen and goes down into the thigh. The femoral artery starts as a continuation of the external iliac artery which comes from the abdominal aorta. The femoral artery is first known as the common femoral artery, because it has not yet given off branches. It gives off a branch known as the deep artery of the thigh (profunda femoris) while continuing down the thigh along the femur. After giving off other branches, the femoral artery goes behind the knee and becomes the popliteal artery.

Informed Consent

Consent by a patient to a surgical or medical procedure or participation in a clinical study after achieving an understanding of the relevant medical facts and the risks involved.

Injury

Damage or harm done to or suffered by a person or thing; a particular form of hurt, damage, or loss; Violation of the rights of another party for which legal redress is available.

Insufflate

To treat medically by blowing a powder, gas, or vapor into a bodily cavity.

Insurance

Coverage by a contract binding a party to indemnify another against specified loss in return for premiums paid.

Interrogatories

A formal or written question, as to a witness, usually requiring a response or answer under oath.

Judgment

A determination of a court of law; a judicial decision.

Jurisdiction

The right and power to interpret and apply the law: *courts having jurisdiction in this district.*

Laparoscopy

A type of minimally invasive surgery in which a small incision (cut) is made in the abdominal wall through which an instrument called a laparoscope is inserted to permit structures within the abdomen and pelvis to be seen. The abdominal cavity is distended and made visible by the instillation of absorbable gas, typically, carbon dioxide. A diversity of tubes can be pushed through the same incision in the skin. Probes or other instruments can thus be introduced through the same opening. In this way, several surgical procedures can be performed without the need for a large surgical incision. Most patients receive general anesthesia during the procedure. The advantages of laparoscopy include a shorter post-operative period with less pain. The avoidance of a large abdominal incision also decreases some of the post-op complications related to the heart and lungs. In addition, there is decreased mortality with some laparoscopic procedures, as compared to the old open surgical procedures.

Laparotomy

A surgical incision into the abdominal wall, often done to examine abdominal organs.

Lawsuit

An action brought in a court for the purpose of seeking relief from or remedy for an alleged wrong.

Lawyer

See *Attorney*.

Liable

Legally obligated or responsible.

Litigation

To contest or engage in legal proceedings.

Malpractice

Improper or negligent treatment of a patient, as by a physician, resulting in injury, damage, or loss; negligence, misconduct, lack of ordinary skill, or a breach of duty in the performance of a professional service resulting in injury or loss.

Mediation

An attempt to bring about a peaceful settlement or compromise between disputants through the objective intervention of a neutral party.

Mediator

A negotiator who acts as a link between parties; one that works to effect reconciliation, settlement, or compromise between parties at variance.

Medical Code of Silence

The practice in which doctors resist testifying against other doctors, medical practitioners or medical institutions.

Medical Records

A chronological written account of a patient's examination and treatment that includes the patient's medical history and complaints, the physician's physical findings, the results of diagnostic tests and procedures, and medications and therapeutic procedures.

Misconduct

When doctors provide substandard care or behave unethically or unprofessionally, ranging from improper diagnosis, medication errors and surgical mistakes to physical and/or sexual assault.

Mitigate

To lessen or minimize the severity of one's losses or damage; lessen or to try to lessen the seriousness or extent of.

Negligence

Failure to exercise the degree of care considered reasonable under the circumstances, resulting in an unintended injury to another party.

OB/GYN

A commonly used abbreviation. OB is short for obstetrics or for an obstetrician, a physician who delivers babies. GYN is short for gynecology or for a gynecologist, a physician who specializes in treating diseases of the female reproductive organs. The word "gynecology" comes from the Greek *gyno, gynaikos* meaning woman + logia meaning study, so gynecology literally is the study of women. Today, gynecology is focused largely on disorders of the female reproductive organs. An obstetrician/gynecologist (OB/GYN) is therefore a physician who both delivers babies and treats diseases of the female reproductive organs.

Obstetrics

See OB/GYN.

Operative Report

A part of a patient's medical record, written or dictated by the physician who played a specific role in a greater portion of a patient's medical treatment.

Pain and Suffering

Mental or especially physical distress for which one may seek damages in a tort action.

Petition

> A formal written application requesting a court for a specific judicial action.

Physician

> A skilled health-care professional trained and licensed to practice medicine.

Plaintiff

> A person who brings an action in a court of law or the party that institutes a suit in a court.

Practitioner

> One who practices medicine or an allied health profession.

Prayer Chain

> A team or network of Christians mobilized to pray for a common cause.

Proceedings

> A course of action; a procedure, or the institution of a sequence of steps by which legal judgments are invoked.

Psychologist

> A specialist in one or more branches of psychology; a practitioner of clinical psychology, counseling, or guidance.

Request for Production

> A discovery request served by one party to an action on another for the presentation for inspection of specified documents or tangible things or for permission to enter upon and inspect property in the other party's possession.

Res ipsa loquitor

Latin term meaning, *the thing speaks for itself*: A doctrine or rule of evidence in tort law that permits an inference or presumption that a defendant was negligent in an accident injuring the plaintiff on the basis of circumstantial evidence if the accident was of a kind that does not ordinarily occur in the absence of negligence.

Respondeat superior

Latin term meaning, *let the superior give answer*: a doctrine in tort law that makes a master liable for the wrong of a servant; *specifically*: the doctrine making an employer or principal liable for the wrong of an employee or agent if it was committed within the scope of employment or agency.

Resuscitation

Act of reviving a person and returning them to consciousness; to restore consciousness, vigor, or life to.

Specialist

A physician whose practice is limited to a particular branch of medicine or surgery, especially one who is certified by a board of physicians.

Spirometer

An instrument for measuring the volume of air entering and leaving the lungs.

Statute of Limitations

A statute setting a time limit on legal action in certain cases; it establishes a period of time from the accrual of a cause of action (as upon the occurrence or discovery of an injury) within which a right of action must be exercised.

Subclavian Artery

A part of a major artery of the upper extremities or forelimbs that passes beneath the clavicle and is continuous with the axillary artery; either of two arteries that supply blood to the neck and arms.

Summons

A call by an authority to appear, come, or do something; a notice summoning a defendant to appear in court, or a notice summoning a person to report to court as a juror or witness.

Tort

Damage, injury, or a wrongful act done willfully, negligently, or in circumstances involving strict liability, but not involving breach of contract, for which a civil suit can be brought.

Tort Reform

A modern movement or political effort to limit jury awards to plaintiffs in medical malpractice lawsuits, based upon the belief that restricting these awards will result in lower medical costs and reduce frivolous lawsuits.

Transcript

Something that has been transcribed; a written record (usually typewritten) of dictated or recorded speech; a reproduction of a written record.

Transfusion

The introduction of blood or blood plasma into a vein or artery; the process of transfusing fluid into a vein or artery.

Trocar

A sharp-pointed surgical instrument, used with a cannula to puncture a body cavity for fluid aspiration or fluid drainage outlet.

Vascular Surgeon

A medical specialist that specializes in performing surgical procedures pertaining to the blood vessels.

Vena cava

The superior vena cava is the large vein which returns blood to the heart from the head, neck and both upper limbs. The inferior vena cava returns blood to the heart from the lower part of the body. The superior vena cava is located in the middle of the chest and is surrounded by rigid structures and lymph nodes.

Verdict

The finding of a jury in a trial.